T0226907

Osteoporosis and Fragility Fractures

Editors

JASON A. LOWE
GARY E. FRIEDLAENDER

ORTHOPEDIC CLINICS OF NORTH AMERICA

www.orthopedic.theclinics.com

April 2013 • Volume 44 • Number 2

ELSEVIER

1600 John F. Kennedy Boulevard • Suite 1800 • Philadelphia, Pennsylvania, 19103-2899.

http://www.theclinics.com

ORTHOPEDIC CLINICS OF NORTH AMERICA Volume 44, Number 2
April 2013 ISSN 0030-5898, ISBN-13: 978-1-4557-7131-8

Editor: Jessica McCool
Developmental Editor: Teia Stone

© **2013 Elsevier Inc. All rights reserved.**

This journal and the individual contributions contained in it are protected under copyright by Elsevier, and the following terms and conditions apply to their use:

Photocopying
Single photocopies of single articles may be made for personal use as allowed by national copyright laws. Permission of the Publisher and payment of a fee is required for all other photocopying, including multiple or systematic copying, copying for advertising or promotional purposes, resale, and all forms of document delivery. Special rates are available for educational institutions that wish to make photocopies for non-profit educational classroom use. For information on how to seek permission visit www.elsevier.com/permissions or call: (+44) 1865 843830 (UK)/(+1) 215 239 3804 (USA).

Derivative Works
Subscribers may reproduce tables of contents or prepare lists of articles including abstracts for internal circulation within their institutions. Permission of the Publisher is required for resale or distribution outside the institution. Permission of the Publisher is required for all other derivative works, including compilations and translations (please consult www.elsevier.com/permissions).

Electronic Storage or Usage
Permission of the Publisher is required to store or use electronically any material contained in this journal, including any article or part of an article (please consult www.elsevier.com/permissions). Except as outlined above, no part of this publication may be reproduced, stored in a retrieval system or transmitted in any form or by any means, electronic, mechanical, photocopying, recording or otherwise, without prior written permission of the Publisher.

Notice
No responsibility is assumed by the Publisher for any injury and/or damage to persons or property as a matter of products liability, negligence or otherwise, or from any use or operation of any methods, products, instructions or ideas contained in the material herein. Because of rapid advances in the medical sciences, in particular, independent verification of diagnoses and drug dosages should be made.

Although all advertising material is expected to conform to ethical (medical) standards, inclusion in this publication does not constitute a guarantee or endorsement of the quality or value of such product or of the claims made of it by its manufacturer.

Orthopedic Clinics of North America (ISSN 0030-5898) is published quarterly by Elsevier Inc., 360 Park Avenue South, New York, NY 10010-1710. Months of issue are January, April, July, and October. Business and Editorial Offices: 1600 John F. Kennedy Blvd., Suite 1800, Philadelphia, PA 19103-2899. Customer Service Office: 3251 Riverport Lane, Maryland Heights, MO 63043. Periodicals postage paid at New York, NY and additional mailing offices. Subscription prices are $293.00 per year for (US individuals), $554.00 per year for (US institutions), $347.00 per year (Canadian individuals), $664.00 per year (Canadian institutions), $427.00 per year (international individuals), $689.00 per year (international institutions), $144.00 per year (US students), $208.00 per year (Canadian and international students). Foreign air speed delivery is included in all *Clinics* subscription prices. All prices are subject to change without notice. **POSTMASTER:** Send change of address to *Orthopedic Clinics of North America*, **Elsevier Health Sciences Division, Subscription Customer Service, 3251 Riverport Lane, Maryland Heights, MO 63043. Customer Service (orders, claims, online, change of address): Elsevier Health Sciences Division, Subscription Customer Service, 3251 Riverport Lane, Maryland Heights, MO 63043. Tel: 1-800-654-2452 (U.S. and Canada); 314-447-8871 (outside U.S. and Canada). Fax: 314-447-8029. E-mail: journalscustomerservice-usa@elsevier. com (for print support); journalsonlinesupport-usa@elsevier.com (for online support).**

Reprints. For copies of 100 or more, of articles in this publication, please contact the Commercial Reprints Department, Elsevier Inc., 360 Park Avenue South, New York, NY 10010-1710. Tel.: 212-633-3812; Fax: 212-462-1935; E-mail: reprints@elsevier. com.

Orthopedic Clinics of North America is covered in *MEDLINE/PubMed* (*Index Medicus*), *Cinahl, Excerpta Medica,* and *Cumulative Index to Nursing and Allied Health Literature.*

Printed and bound by CPI Group (UK) Ltd, Croydon, CR0 4YY

Transferred to digital print 2013

Contributors

EDITORS

JASON A. LOWE, MD
Assistant Professor, Orthopaedic Trauma
Surgery, Director, Fragility Fracture Program,
University of Alabama at Birmingham,
Birmingham, Alabama

GARY E. FRIEDLAENDER, MD
Professor of Orthopedics and Rehabilitation,
Yale University School of Medicine,
New Haven, Connecticut

AUTHORS

MICHAEL R. BAUMGAERTNER, MD
Professor of Orthopaedics and Rehabilitation,
Director of Orthopaedic Trauma, Department
of Orthopaedics and Rehabilitation, Yale
University School of Medicine, New Haven,
Connecticut

JUDITH F. BAUMHAUER, MD, MPH
Professor and Associate Chair of Academic
Affairs, Department of Orthopaedics and
Rehabilitation, University of Rochester Medical
Center, Rochester, New York; President,
American Orthopaedic Foot and Ankle Society,
Rosemont, Illinois

MOHIT BHANDARI, MD, PhD, FRCSC
Division of Orthopaedic Surgery, McMaster
University, Hamilton, Ontario, Canada

LJILJANA BOGUNOVIC, MD
Resident, Department of Orthopedic Surgery,
Washington University, St Louis, Missouri

HARMAN CHAUDHRY, MD
Division of Orthopaedic Surgery, McMaster
University, Hamilton, Ontario, Canada

STEVEN M. CHERNEY, MD
Resident, Department of Orthopedic Surgery,
Washington University, St Louis, Missouri

BRETT D. CRIST, MD, FACS
Associate Professor, Department of
Orthopaedic Surgery, University of Missouri,
Columbia, Missouri

**GREGORY J. DELLA ROCCA, MD,
PhD, FACS**
Associate Professor, Department of
Orthopaedic Surgery, University of Missouri,
Columbia, Missouri

PHILIP J. DEVEREAUX, MD, PhD, FRCPC
Departments of Clinical Epidemiology and
Biostatistics and Medicine, McMaster
University, Hamilton, Ontario, Canada

SHAH-NAWAZ M. DODWAD, MD
Department of Orthopaedics, The Ohio State
University, Columbus, Ohio

MICHAEL J. GARDNER, MD
Resident, Assistant Professor of Orthopedic
Surgery, Department of Orthopedic Surgery,
Washington University, St Louis, Missouri

VISHAL V. HEGDE, BA
Medical student, Weill Cornell Medical College,
Cornell University, New York, New York

PATRICK D.G. HENRY, MD, FRCSC
Clinical Associate, Division of Orthopaedics,
Department of Surgery, Sunnybrook Health
Science Centre, University of Toronto, Toronto,
Ontario, Canada

BRYON HOBBY, MD
Clinical Instructor, Department of Orthopaedic
Surgery, University of California Davis,
Sacramento, California

JOSHUA HUNTER, MD
Resident, Department of Orthopaedics and
Rehabilitation, University of Rochester Medical
Center, Rochester, New York

**RICHARD J. JENKINSON, MD, MPH,
MSc, FRCSC**
Assistant Professor, Division of Orthopaedics,
Department of Surgery, Sunnybrook Health
Science Centre, University of Toronto, Toronto,
Ontario, Canada

SAFDAR N. KHAN, MD
Department of Orthopaedics, The Ohio State
University, Columbus, Ohio

HANS J. KREDER, MD, MPH, FRCSC
Professor, Orthopaedic Surgery and Health
Policy Evaluation and Management, Chief of
Holland Musculoskeletal Program, Marvin Tile
Chair and Chief, Division of Orthopaedic
Surgery, Chair of Medical Advisory Committee,
Sunnybrook Health Science Centre, University
of Toronto, Toronto, Ontario, Canada

JOSEPH M. LANE, MD
Chief, Department of Orthopaedic Surgery,
Hospital for Special Surgery, New York,
New York

MARK A. LEE, MD
Associate Professor, Director, Orthopaedic
Trauma Fellowship, Department of
Orthopaedic Surgery, University of California
Davis, Sacramento, California

MICHAEL P. LESLIE, DO
Assistant Professor of Orthopaedics and
Rehabilitation, Department of Orthopaedics
and Rehabilitation, Yale University School of
Medicine, New Haven, Connecticut

JOSHUA R. OLSEN, MD
Resident, Department of Orthopaedics and
Rehabilitation, University of Rochester Medical
Center, Rochester, New York

ANISH G. POTTY, MD
Orthopaedic Fellow, Department of
Orthopaedic Surgery, Hospital for Special
Surgery, New York, New York

MARCUS A. ROTHERMICH, MD
Resident, Department of Orthopedic Surgery,
Washington University, St Louis, Missouri

KENNETH G. SAAG, MD, MSc
Jane Knight Lowe Professor of Medicine,
Division of Clinical Immunology and
Rheumatology, Department of Medicine,
University of Alabama at Birmingham,
Birmingham, Alabama

ANAS SALEH, MD
Research Fellow, Department of Orthopaedic
Surgery, Hospital for Special Surgery,
New York, New York

AMY H. WARRINER, MD
Assistant Professor, Division of Endocrinology,
Diabetes and Metabolism, Department of
Medicine, University of Alabama at
Birmingham, Birmingham, Alabama

Contents

geriatricians and interdisciplinary care pathways, while continuing to focus on rapid surgical treatment.

The incidence of osteoporotic fractures has been steadily rising along with the aging of the population. Surgical management of these fractures can be a challenge to orthopedic surgeons. Diminished bone mass and frequent comminution make fixation difficult. Advancements in implant design and fixation techniques have served to address these challenges and when properly applied, can improve overall outcome. The purpose of this review is to describe fixation challenges of common osteoporotic fractures and provide options for successful treatment.

Fractures of the acetabulum are some of the most challenging fractures that face orthopedic surgeons. In geriatric patients, these challenges are enhanced by the complexity of fracture patterns, the poor biomechanical characteristics of osteoporotic bone, and the comorbidities present in this population. Nonsurgical management is preferable when the fracture is stable enough to allow mobilization, and healing in a functional position can be expected. When significant displacement and/or hip instability are present, operative management is preferred in most patients, which may include open reduction and internal fixation with or without total hip arthroplasty.

As with most fractures associated with osteoporosis, the incidence of pelvic ring injuries in this population of patients is rising rapidly. Osteoporotic pelvic ring injuries are exceedingly different in their etiology, natural history, and treatment from the more recognizable patterns in young patients with high-energy pelvic ring injuries. Recognition of a potentially unstable fracture pattern, careful evaluation of the ambulatory and functional status of each patient before injury, and the potential pitfalls and benefits of operative versus nonoperative care are critical to the effective treatment.

Ankle fractures are one of the most common injuries in the elderly and their incidence is anticipated to increase over the next 20 years. Appropriate management of ankle fractures in this population requires an understanding of the issues unique to the elderly. Osteoporosis must be considered when counseling patients about their ankle fracture. Good outcomes can be achieved with surgical fixation of ankle fractures in the elderly. Postoperative complications are higher in patients with diabetes and peripheral vascular disease, and in patients who smoke. This article reviews how to evaluate and treat ankle fractures in elderly patients with osteoporosis, evaluates the outcomes, and discusses surgical techniques.

Osteoporosis affects millions of US citizens, and millions more are at risk for developing the disease. Several operative techniques are available to the spine surgeon to provide care for those affected by osteoporosis. The types of osteoporosis, common surgical complications, medical optimization, and surgical techniques in the osteoporotic spine are reviewed, with an emphasis on preoperative planning.

Osteoporosis is a systemic disease that affects millions of people worldwide. It is estimated that 50% of women and approximately 20% of men more than 50 years of age will sustain a fragility fracture. The cause of nonunion in patients with osteoporosis is likely multifactorial, and includes age-related changes in fracture repair as well as challenges in achieving stable internal fixation. This article discusses fracture healing in patients with osteoporosis and the principles of fixation. Pharmacotherapy for the patient with osteoporosis is also discussed.

ORTHOPEDIC CLINICS OF NORTH AMERICA

FORTHCOMING ISSUES

Beginning with the July 2013 issue, *Orthopedic Clinics of North America* will adopt a new format. Rather than focusing on a single topic, each issue will contain articles on key areas in orthopedics—adult reconstruction, upper extremity, trauma, and sports medicine. Articles on pediatrics, oncology, and foot and ankle will also be included on a regular basis. As the practice of orthopedics has become more specialized, the format of one topic per issue is no longer fulfilling our readers' needs. The new format is intended to address these changing needs.

Orthopedic Clinics of North America will continue to publish a print issue four times a year, in January, April, July, and October. However, it will also include online-only articles that will be published on a rolling basis (not in accordance with our quarterly publication dates). These articles, along with articles from our print issues, will be available on http://www.orthopedic.theclinics.com/

RECENT ISSUES

January 2013
Emerging Concepts in Upper Extremity Trauma
Michael P. Leslie, DO and Seth D. Dodds, MD, *Editors*

October 2012
Management of Compressive Neuropathies of the Upper Extremity
Asif M. Ilyas, MD, *Editor*

July 2012
Hip Dysplasia Surgery: Birth to Adulthood
George J. Haidukewych, MD, and
Ernest L. Sinke, MD, *Editors*

ISSUE OF RELATED INTEREST

Endocrinology and Metabolism Clinics of North America,
September 2012 (Vol. 41, Issue 3)
Osteoporosis
Sol Epstein, MD, *Editor*
http://www.endo.theclinics.com/

NOW AVAILABLE FOR YOUR iPhone and iPad

Preface
Osteoporosis and Fragility Fractures

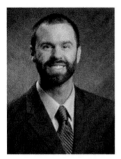
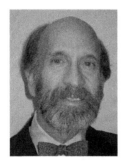

Jason A. Lowe, MD   Gary E. Friedlaender, MD

Editors

The world's demographics are changing. In North America, the fastest growing segment of the population is over 65 years of age. While age is not the only determinant of osteoporosis or general bone health, longevity correlates in a highly reliable manner with diminishing bone mineral density. Osteoporosis (and osteopenia) often begins as a silent condition that, over time, is responsible for a variety of low-energy fragility fractures. These fractures, most typically of the hip region, distal radius, ankle, pelvis, and vertebrae, bring with them special challenges with respect to their biology, biomechanical considerations, fixation requirements, and rehabilitation. General health of patients of advancing age and diminishing bone mass, and their rehabilitation potential, add to the complexity of their care and impact the quality of their treatment outcomes.

In this issue, we have chosen a panel of thoughtful and talented orthopedic surgeons and clinician-scientists to discuss the pathophysiology of osteoporosis, its medical management and the impact of common comordid conditions, fracture repair. We have further asked our contributors to describe important aspects and considerations in the surgical approaches to the most common fragility fractures, especially as they reflect choices of implants and their fixation.

With the increasing incidence of fragility fractures, greater focus and responsibility are being placed on orthopedic surgeons to diagnose and treat osteoporosis. The Joint Commission has stated that "It's time for a change in how osteoporosis is prevented, detected, and treated."[1] The diagnosis and treatment of this "Medical" condition must become the responsibility of all orthopedic surgeons. We must be aware and knowledgable about the biology of osteoporosis and the impact this disorder has on operative management of fragility fractures and the rehabilitation of affected patients. Successful surgical outcomes for osteoporotic patients can be more challenging to achieve than in younger patients, reflecting the geriatric patient's medical frailty

Orthop Clin N Am 44 (2013) ix–x
http://dx.doi.org/10.1016/j.ocl.2013.01.004
0030-5898/13/$ – see front matter © 2013 Published by Elsevier Inc.

and the compromised biological and biomechanical character of their bone.

Most health care professionals will encounter the medically frail geriatric patient. Orthopedic surgeons will be no exception, and it is incumbent on us to be prepared to effectively participate in the management of this important and expanding group of patients, with their special and specific set of circumstances.

Jason A. Lowe, MD
Orthopaedic Trauma Surgery
Fragility Fracture Program
University of Alabama at Birmingham
FOT 901, 510 20th street south
Birmingham, AL 35294, USA

Gary E. Friedlaender, MD
Wayne O. Southwick Professor and Chair
Orthopedics and Rehabilitation
Yale University School of Medicine
P.O. Box 208071
New Haven, CT 06520-8071, USA

E-mail addresses:
jasonlowe@uabmc.edu (J.A. Lowe)
gary.friedlaender@yale.edu (G.E. Friedlaender)

REFERENCE

1. The Joint Commission. Improving and measuring osteoporosis management. Oakbrook Terrace, IL: The Joint Commission; 2007.

Osteoporosis Diagnosis and Medical Treatment

Amy H. Warriner, MD[a],*, Kenneth G. Saag, MD, MSc[b]

KEYWORDS

- Osteoporosis • Treatment • Prevention • Diagnosis • Update

KEY POINTS

- Osteoporosis can be diagnosed by measurement of bone mineral density or based on the history of a nontraumatic fracture.
- Osteoporosis treatment should be considered in all people with an increased risk of future fracture. Use of fracture risk assessment tools can assist in determining patients who would benefit from treatment.
- There are several therapies available for the treatment and prevention of osteoporosis. The optimal treatment option for each patient should be determined after weighing the benefits and potential risks associated with these medications.
- Further information is needed to assist clinicians in determining the duration of osteoporosis treatment and the potential role of an interrupted treatment regimen.

INTRODUCTION

Hip fractures and vertebral fractures are 2 of the most common fracture sites related to osteoporosis, and affect nearly 1 million persons in the United States annually.[1] Moreover, nearly one-quarter of patients who endure a hip fracture die within a year of the fracture. An even larger proportion requires either extensive physical rehabilitation or a stay in a nursing home facility. In addition to the morbidity and mortality patients may experience after an osteoporotic fracture, there are significant health care costs associated with fractures. The estimated cost of osteoporosis-related fractures in 2005 was $19 billion, but this is estimated to increase to more than $25 billion per year in the next 2 decades.[1,2] However, many of these fractures could be prevented if osteoporosis and fracture risk were assessed before a fracture and appropriate measures taken.

DEFINITION OF OSTEOPOROSIS

Osteoporosis can be defined clinically by either:

1. Low bone mineral density (BMD) (T-score of ≤ -2.5)
2. A history of fragility fracture

BMD is measured by a central dual-energy x-ray absorptiometry (DXA) scan. BMD is presented as gram per centimeter squared, then translated into T-scores for postmenopausal women and men older than 50 years. Alternatively, Z-scores are used for premenopausal women and younger men. T-scores and Z-scores represent the patient's BMD in relation to a 30-year-old normal reference and an age-matched reference, respectively, and the difference is presented as a standard deviation from the "normal" BMD. The World Health Organization (WHO) defines osteoporosis as a T-score of -2.5 and lower; osteopenia (or low bone density)

Disclosures: [A.W.] Research: Amylin; [K.G.S.] Research and/or consulting: Amgen, Eli Lilly, Merck, Novartis.
[a] Division of Endocrinology, Metabolism and Diabetes, University of Alabama at Birmingham, 2000 6th Avenue South, FOT 702, Birmingham, AL 35233, USA; [b] Division of Clinical Immunology and Rheumatology, University of Alabama at Birmingham, 2000 6th Avenue South, FOT 702, Birmingham, AL 35233, USA
* Corresponding author.
E-mail address: warriner@uab.edu

Orthop Clin N Am 44 (2013) 125–135
http://dx.doi.org/10.1016/j.ocl.2013.01.005
0030-5898/13/$ – see front matter © 2013 Elsevier Inc. All rights reserved.

orthopedic.theclinics.com

as a T-score between −1.0 and −2.5; and normal bone density as a T-score of −1.0 and higher. In a younger population, Z-scores of −2.0 and lower reflect low BMD and any Z-score higher than −2.0 is normal.

Based on the WHO definition, osteoporosis can also be diagnosed based on a prior "osteoporotic" fracture. Other ways of describing an osteoporotic fracture include fractures that would not have typically occurred in a "normal" individual, or a "fragility fracture." Fragility fracture is frequently described as a fracture occurring as the result of minimal trauma or a fall from standing height or less. All of these definitions are subjective and leave room for clinical judgment. A history of hip or vertebral fracture is sufficient for a diagnosis of osteoporosis and recommendation for treatment regardless of BMD,[1] but most other prior fractures also convey an increased risk of future fracture.[3] However, fractures in adults are commonly managed without consideration of future risk. Thus, the American Orthopaedic Association launched the "Own the Bone" program in 2009 in an effort to increase the awareness of fragility fractures as a teachable moment. The intent of the program is recognition of patients who have an initial fracture and to ensure that they have proper evaluation for osteoporosis and treatment where appropriate.

There is intentional movement away from the T-scores alone, which measure relative fracture risk, toward absolute fracture risk. The WHO developed a fracture risk assessment tool called FRAX,[4] which allows for the addition of clinical information to BMD (or body mass index, if BMD is not available). FRAX integrates clinical risk factors, such as glucocorticoid use, smoking, alcohol use, family history of fracture, and prior fracture, into the determination of 10-year absolute fracture risk. These estimates of fracture risk can then be used to assist in determining treatment needed in patients with less clear indications or to discuss potential treatment benefits with patients. A similar but more patient-friendly tool called the Garvin Institute Fracture Risk Calculator can be downloaded at http://garvan.org.au/promotions/bone-fracture-risk/calculator/index.php.

OSTEOPOROSIS IN MEN

In contrast to most diseases for which there is a relative abundance of data and emphasis on men's health, the opposite is true for osteoporosis. In 2012, the Endocrine Society published clinical guidelines for the treatment of osteoporosis in men.[5] Based on these guidelines, it is now recommended that all men at risk of osteoporosis or fracture obtain a DXA scan for screening. Based on

age alone, men who are 70 years or older should undergo screening. In addition, men aged 50 to 69 should also undergo DXA evaluation if additional risk factors for osteoporosis are present (**Table 1**). Based on the DXA findings, men with T-scores in the osteoporosis range or men with low BMD and other clinical risk factors for fracture should be initiated on an osteoporosis prescription medication.

It is estimated that 30% to 60% of osteoporosis within men is secondary to another underlying condition.[6] The most frequent secondary causes are glucocorticoid use or hypercortisolism (ie, Cushing syndrome or disease), excessive alcohol use, hypogonadism, vitamin D deficiency/low calcium intake, smoking, and family history of fracture. Other secondary causes combined account for approximately 15% of cases. In up to 40% of cases in men no secondary cause is identified, and the osteoporosis is considered either primary or idiopathic osteoporosis.[6] Secondary causes (see **Table 1**) for osteoporosis and fracture should be assessed clinically (by history and physical examination) in all patients, and with laboratory evaluation when clinical suspicion is high. Treatment of secondary causes of osteoporosis is recommended. However, if a patient's risk of fracture is high, pharmacologic osteoporosis treatment should be initiated as well. In lower-risk

Table 1 Secondary causes of osteoporosis	
Men and women	Hyperparathyroidism
	Untreated thyroid disease
	Chronic lung disease
	Chronic glucocorticoid use (>3 mo)
	Alcohol abuse (>3 alcoholic beverages daily)
	Smoking tobacco use
	Vitamin D insufficiency
	Low calcium intake
	Immobilization
	Anorexia nervosa
	Diabetes mellitus (types 1 and 2)
	Adrenal insufficiency
	Malabsorptive gastrointestinal disease (celiac, inflammatory bowel disease, gastric bypass, etc)
	Rheumatoid arthritis
	Systemic lupus erythematosus
	Ankylosing spondylitis
Men	Hypogonadism
	Gonadotropin-releasing hormone agonist treatment
Women	Ovarian failure
	Amenorrhea (hypogonadotropic hypogonadism)

patients treatment of the secondary cause may be sufficient, but they should be monitored for future bone loss and fracture risk.

RISK OF FUTURE FRACTURE
Prior Fracture

Low-energy trauma fractures have historically been linked to osteoporosis, in part because of the increased risk of ensuing low-energy fractures. In one study, an increased risk of subsequent fracture was observed following any fragility fracture, with only 2 exceptions: rib fractures in men and ankle fractures in women.[7] In a more recent study nearly all fragility fractures were significantly associated with future fracture among postmenopausal women.[3] In this study, ankle fractures were associated with an increased risk of future fracture of weight-bearing bones and rib fractures were associated with a risk of future vertebral fracture. Of note, the associations between incident hip and vertebral fracture following prior hip and vertebral fractures, respectively, were significantly elevated (hazard ratio [HR] of 7.3 and 3.5, respectively).

In addition to findings that most fracture types increase the risk of future fracture, there is also evidence that even fractures associated with high-energy trauma pose a risk for future fracture.[8,9] Several studies have shown that BMD is similar in those who have had prior fractures, regardless of the presence or absence of high-energy trauma. In several studies, individuals with fractures were 3 times more likely to have osteoporosis at 1 or more sites regardless of the degree of trauma at the time of fracture.[10–12] It has also been shown that a relationship exists between high-trauma fractures and either low BMD or structural changes in bone in both women and men, comparable with the relationship seen in those who have had low-energy trauma fractures.[9,10,13] These findings all suggest that any prior fracture as an adult (after age 50 years), regardless of the degree of trauma, may merit evaluation for underlying fragility and may be associated with an increased risk of future fracture.

FRACTURE PREVENTION
Nonpharmacologic Treatment Options

Approximately 90% of hip fractures are caused by falls.[14] Several modifiable factors that may mitigate the risk of a fall include a home-safety assessment, alcohol cessation, vision evaluation, medication review (specifically psychoactive medications), and assessment of orthostatic blood pressure. Studies of community dwellers have shown a significant reduction of falls and fractures following exercise intervention.[15–21]

Direction of fall is an important predictor of hip fracture,[22] lending support to the use of hip protectors. Hip protectors significantly reduce the force to the hip during a fall.[23] A meta-analysis showed a slight reduction in the risk of hip fracture among nursing home or residential care patients randomized to a hip protector (relative risk [RR] 0.77, 95% confidence interval [CI] 0.62–0.97) but no significant benefit among community dwellers was found (RR 1.16, 95% CI 0.85–1.59). The differences may be explained by poor long-term adherence in both patient groups, and should be interpreted cautiously because of cluster randomization.[24] Another trial randomized individual nursing home residents to a one-sided hip protector and, despite good adherence, found no reduction in hip fractures in the unprotected versus protected hip.[25] Despite these inconsistent results, hip protectors may still be a safe and reasonable option.

Calcium and vitamin D

Randomized trials comparing calcium therapy alone versus placebo have shown no consistent benefit in the reduction of vertebral and nonvertebral fractures.[26–29] These findings may be partially confounded by nonadherence with treatment, because other trials have shown that when adherence of 80% or better is achieved, calcium has been shown to reduce the risk of fracture (HR 0.66, 95% CI 0.45–0.97).[27]

Most available studies of calcium are completed in combination with vitamin D supplementation. Although there is evidence that calcium and vitamin D reduce the risk of fracture, the benefit has not been seen in all populations.[30–38] The type and amount of vitamin D supplementation likely play a role in the reduction of fracture risk.[37]

Evidence associating vitamin D intake with fracture reduction exists. In a meta-analysis, oral vitamin D supplementation of any dose led to a 7% to 10% reduction of fracture risk in older people (HR for any nonvertebral fracture 0.93, 95% CI, 0.87–0.99; HR for hip fracture 0.90, 95% CI 0.80–1.01).[39] However, in those subjects who took the highest vitamin D doses (median of 800 IU/d), the reduction of fracture risk was greater (HR for any nonvertebral fracture 0.70, 95% CI 0.58–0.86; HR for hip fracture 0.86, 95% CI 0.76–0.96). These data underscore the importance of the dose when recommending vitamin D supplementation.

In addition to its role in fracture reduction, vitamin D insufficiency has been found to be associated with risk of a fall[40] and supplementation has been found to reduce the risk of falls, likely through improved musculoskeletal function.[41–43] Two randomized clinical trials confirmed that vitamin D supplementation (cholecalciferol 700 IU daily) reduced the risk of a fall in elderly persons.[44,45] The effect was shown even in persons with adequate 25-hydroxyvitamin D (25(OH)D) levels at the start of the study,[44,45] and was found to be more prominent in the less active women studied.[44] The US Preventive Services Task Force has recently published recommendations for fall prevention in older, community-dwelling adults, which include vitamin D supplementation along with exercise for fall prevention.[46]

Vitamin D is important in bone health because of its ability to counterregulate parathyroid hormone (PTH), a promoter of bone loss, and its ability to stimulate intestinal and renal calcium absorption. In the setting of vitamin D deficiency, PTH levels typically increase, resulting in secondary hyperparathyroidism.

The optimal level of serum 25(OH)D remains unclear, as do the optimal doses of vitamin D for replacement and maintenance. Most agree that vitamin D deficiency can be defined as a 25(OH)D level of less than 20 ng/mL.[47] Because a 25(OH)D level of less than 30 ng/mL is sometimes associated with PTH elevation, a serum 25(OH)D level of 30 ng/mL has been recommended by some.[48,49] Vitamin D intoxication, leading to hypercalcemia, generally does not occur until 25(OH)D levels reach 150 ng/mL or higher, except in patients with primary hyperparathyroidism.[47,50,51]

Because of the multiple confounders regarding the absolute benefit of calcium, it is recommended that persons take calcium and vitamin D supplements for general bone health but that these supplements should not be used alone for the reduction of fracture risk. The Institute of Medicine published recommendations for calcium and vitamin D usage in 2011 based on age and gender

(**Table 2**).[52] These new recommendations state that women 51 years and older and men 71 years and older should aim to consume 1200 mg of calcium daily, whereas a daily intake of 1000 mg is recommended for women 19 to 50 and men 19 to 70 years of age. For vitamin D, the recommended daily intake is 600 IU daily for children and adults, but rises to a recommended dose of 800 IU daily for men and women 71 years and older.

Shortly after the recommendations from the Institute of Medicine were published, the Endocrine Society published recommendations for vitamin D dosing provided by an expert committee (see **Table 2**)[53]. In these latter recommendations, the recommended daily intake of vitamin D was much higher (1500–2000 IU daily for men and women) than that proposed by the Institute of Medicine.

A concern has been raised regarding a potential association between calcium and vitamin D supplementation and cardiovascular risk.[54–57] In a secondary analysis of a prospective, placebo-controlled study of calcium supplementation in postmenopausal women, an association between calcium supplements and myocardial infarction and composite cardiovascular disease was seen, but was attenuated after the addition of unreported cardiovascular events found in the national hospital admission database.[57] Thereafter, meta-analyses also found an association between calcium supplements alone and increased cardiovascular risk,[56] and this was further supported by the update of this meta-analysis that included calcium with or without concurrent vitamin D.[55] By contrast, another meta-analysis refuted these findings and found no clear association between cardiovascular disease and calcium supplementation.[54] Similarly, in a recent report no association was found between cardiovascular disease and

Table 2
Recommendations from the Institute of Medicine and the Endocrine Society for daily intake of calcium and vitamin D in men and women

| Age (y) | Institute of Medicine[52] | | Endocrine Society[72] | |
	Recommended Daily Allowance	Upper Daily Limit	Daily Requirement	Upper Daily Limit
Calcium (mg)				
19–50	1000	2500	—	—
51–70	1000 (men) 1200 (women)	2000	—	—
>70	1200	2000	—	—
Vitamin D (IU)				
19–70	600	4000	1500–2000	10000
>70	800	4000	1500–2000	10000

calcium supplementation in women enrolled in the Nurses' Health Study, including women taking higher daily doses of calcium (>1000 mg of calcium daily).[58]

Based on these findings, it is appropriate to assess each patient's daily calcium consumption. If a patient is consuming fewer than 3 servings of calcium-rich foods or beverages daily (ie, milk, yogurt, cheese, calcium-fortified orange juice, and so forth), calcium supplementation should be considered. Goal daily calcium intake should be between 1000 and 1500 mg per day, divided. Care should be taken to avoid oversupplementation because of the risk of nephrolithiasis and, potentially, cardiovascular disease. Unlike calcium, vitamin D is more difficult to obtain from common foods and beverages. Patients older than 70 years are also less likely to obtain adequate vitamin D through sun exposure. Therefore, supplementation is typically required. The recommended daily intake of vitamin D is a minimum of 800 IU daily, but many patients require 1000 to 2000 IU daily to maintain stores of vitamin D.

Pharmacologic Treatment Options

The initial question most clinicians have is: who should be treated? The second question is determining which treatment to begin. The National Osteoporosis Foundation has created some guidelines to assist with the first question (**Box 1**), which rely on data obtained through imaging (DXA) and/or clinical risk factors for fracture. As such, a DXA is not essential in determining the need for treatment. Consequently, in a patient with a recent hip, vertebral, or other weight-bearing osteoporotic fracture, treatment should be initiated without the need for BMD measurement, if no other contraindications exist. Treatment also should be initiated in a patient without a prior fracture but who has other strong clinical risk factors for fracture.

Box 1
Indications for osteoporosis prescription therapy

Hip or vertebral fracture

Osteoporosis based on BMD (T-score ≤ -2.5) after appropriate evaluation for secondary causes

Low bone density by BMD (T-score of -1.0 to -2.5) **and** risk based on the FRAX algorithm (10-year probability of a major osteoporosis-related fracture of $\geq 20\%$ **or** 10-year probability of a hip fracture of $\geq 3\%$)

Clinical judgment based on overall fracture risk

The armamentarium for osteoporosis management is growing. At present, treatment options can be divided into antiresorptive medications and anabolic medications (**Table 3**).

Bisphosphonates

Bisphosphonates are the most commonly prescribed antiosteoporosis medications. These agents inhibit osteoclast function, thereby reducing bone resorption. The bisphosphonates are available as either oral preparations or intravenous infusions. Under ideal conditions orally administered bisphosphonates have a very low estimated absorption of 1% of the administered dose. Following absorption, the bisphosphonate is integrated into hydroxyapatite.

Alendronate (Fosamax) and risedronate (Actonel) were among the first bisphosphonates approved for the treatment and prevention of osteoporosis in postmenopausal women, and were approved for the treatment of male osteoporosis thereafter. Both can be taken either daily or weekly (see **Table 3**). Risedronate can also be taken in a once-monthly preparation or as a delayed-release weekly preparation that can be taken with food and other medications (Atelvia). Ibandronate (Boniva) is approved for oral use daily or once monthly, or intravenously every 3 months. The main side effect reported with the use of oral bisphosphonates is gastrointestinal intolerance. Oral bisphosphonates have significant reduction of efficacy if not dosed appropriately, owing to its limited absorption (taken on empty stomach with only water and no further oral intake for at least 30–60 minutes, except for Atelvia).

Zoledronic acid (Reclast) is the newest bisphosphonate available, and is a once-yearly intravenous option. In addition to initial trials completed in postmenopausal women, zoledronic acid has also been found to be effective in the prevention of recurrent fractures (over a median follow-up of 1.9 years) based on a large study of patients who received this medication within 90 days of a hip fracture.[59] This study also demonstrated a 28% reduction of mortality risk with the use of this agent compared with placebo, although the potential mechanism for this benefit was unclear. The main side effect noted following zoledronic acid infusions is an acute-phase reaction, consisting of flu-like symptoms and fever. The occurrence of this side effect is reduced in patients who have had prior exposure to other bisphosphonates, and can also be reduced by pretreatment with acetaminophen.

All 4 of the bisphosphonates approved in the United States have been studied in large, randomized controlled trials in postmenopausal

Table 3
Prescription osteoporosis prevention and treatment options approved by the Food and Drug Administration, and estimates of associated reduction in fracture risk

	Recommended Use for Osteoporosis			Effect on Fracture Risk			
	Prevention	Treatment in Women	Treatment in Men	Vertebral	Nonvertebral	Hip	Dosing
Antiresorptive Agents							
Bisphosponates							
Alendronate (Fosamax)[73,74]	✓	✓	✓	✓	✓	✓	70 mg oral weekly
Ibandronate (Boniva)[75,76]	✓	✓	—	✓	—	—	150 mg oral monthly 3 mg IV every 3 mo
Risedronate (Actonel, Atelvia)[77,78]	✓	✓	✓	✓	✓	✓	35 mg oral weekly (Actonel, Atelvia) 75 mg oral 2 consecutive days each month (Actonel only) 150 mg oral monthly (Actonel only)
Zolendronic acid (Reclast)[64,79]	✓	✓	✓	✓	✓	✓	5 mg IV yearly
Denosumab (Prolia)[80,81]	—	✓	✓	✓	✓	✓	60 mg SQ every 6 mo
Calcitonin (Miacalcin, Fortical)[82,83]	—	✓	—	✓	—	—	200 IU intranasally daily
Raloxifene (Evista)[84,85]	✓	✓	—	✓	—	—	60 mg oral daily
Anabolic Agent							
Teriparatide (Forteo)[86,87]	—	✓	✓	✓	✓	—	20 µg SQ daily

Abbreviations: IV, intravenous; SQ, subcutaneous.

women, and have shown efficacy in reducing fracture occurrence and improving BMD, although they vary in the relative reduction of fractures (see **Table 3**). The initial phase III clinical trial of alendronate for the treatment of postmenopausal osteoporosis showed significantly greater gain in BMD at all sites and a 48% reduction in new vertebral fractures when compared with placebo.[60] In a separate study, nonvertebral fracture rates were reduced by 47% in postmenopausal women with low bone density treated with alendronate compared with women treated with placebo.[61] Risedronate was evaluated in a higher-risk population of postmenopausal women with osteoporosis and at least 1 prevalent vertebral fracture.[62] Similar to alendronate, BMD increased significantly at all sites. In addition, new vertebral fracture risk was reduced by 65% and nonvertebral fracture risk was reduced by 39% in this higher-risk population. Ibandronate was evaluated in both a daily dose and an intermittent dose (20 mg every other day for 12 doses every 3 months) in postmenopausal women, and was found to increase spine and hip BMD and also to lead to a vertebral reduction in fracture risk of 62% for daily dosing and 50% for intermittent dosing.[63] Zoledronic acid as an annual intravenous infusion in postmenopausal women was evaluated in comparison with placebo.[64] In this study, morphometric vertebral fractures were reduced by 70%, clinical vertebral fractures were reduced by 77%, hip fractures were reduced by 41%, and nonvertebral fractures were reduced by 15% in the treatment group.

Denosumab

Denosumab is a fully human monoclonal antibody that inhibits receptor activator of nuclear factor κB ligand (RANKL), which is important in the differentiation and activation of osteoclasts. Through this action, denosumab inhibits bone resorption similarly to bisphosphonates but through a different mechanism. Denosumab was approved for use in the treatment of osteoporosis in June 2010. Unlike bisphosphonates that require integration into the bone matrix and can be found within the bone matrix years after administration, denosumab concentrations peak in the first 1 to 3 weeks after administration and then decline over 4 to 5 months, and are near nadir levels at the end of its dosing interval (6 months). Concurrently, levels of bone turnover markers decrease quickly after the administration of denosumab and then begin rising toward pretreatment levels at the end of the dosing interval.[65]

Risks Associated with Antiresorptive Treatments

Concerns about long-term risks have been raised with all antiresorptive medications, namely subtrochanteric femur fractures and osteonecrosis of the jaw. These concerns have led to further discussions on the long-term safety and recommended duration of use. Although many clinicians are recommending "drug holidays" for postmenopausal osteoporosis treatment, there has been no justification for this recommendation through randomized trials. Overall, the absolute risk of subtrochanteric femur fractures and osteonecrosis of the jaw is very small and a clear causative effect has not been found, although accumulating evidence from observational studies clearly suggests a strong association.

Two commentaries on the duration of use of bisphosphonates were published in 2012. In the findings from the Food and Drug Administration (FDA) Advisory Committee for Reproductive Health Drugs and the Drug Safety and Risk Management Committee's review, continuation of a bisphosphonate should be determined based on a patient's risk of fracture and the prior duration of treatment.[66] The committee relied on 3 long-term treatment studies of the bisphosphonates alendronate, risedronate, and zoledronic acid that reported fracture rates in postmenopausal women. Based on post hoc analyses of these studies, it was determined that fracture rates between women continued on bisphosphonates and those who stopped bisphosphonates were relatively similar. Thus, the committee recommends that clinicians consider stopping bisphosphonate treatment after 3 to 5 years in women at lower risk of fracture (no prior fracture, BMD near normal) and continue treatment in women at higher risk of fracture (older women with a history of a fracture and BMD in the osteoporotic range). There currently are no recommendations for when to consider restarting treatment if it is stopped or if there is a finite duration for the use of these medications.

Black and colleagues[67] reanalyzed the original alendronate and zoledronic acid extension studies and determined the numbers needed to treat to prevent future fracture. Based on this information, the investigators reached similar conclusions to those of the FDA but emphasized that these recommendations were for alendronate and zoledronic acid only, because long-term data on risedronate and ibandronate were not assessed or available. Their recommendations were to consider stopping previously prescribed bisphosphonates in women with T-scores better than −2.0 and no prior fracture, as their risk for future vertebral fracture is relatively low. Conversely, women with a history of a fracture and a T-score of −2.5 or lower should be continued on bisphosphonate treatment and, although the data are slightly weaker, women with a T-score of −2.0 to −2.5 and a prior fracture should also continue treatment because of the relatively higher risk of future fracture in these individuals. It is hoped that future studies will lend further understanding of how women whose bisphosphonate has been stopped should be followed.

Anabolic Treatment

Teriparatide (Forteo), recombinant human PTH 1-34, is the only anabolic treatment option for osteoporosis. Intermittent PTH exposure, rather than constant exposure as in primary hyperparathyroidism, results in increased bone mass. The use of teriparatide results in significant improvement of BMD and reduction of vertebral and nonvertebral fracture risk. Teriparatide is administered through a daily subcutaneous injection. It is currently approved for use for those at high risk of fracture and for glucocorticoid-induced osteoporosis.[68] Teriparatide should not be used in children or young patients with open epiphyses, or in persons with Paget disease, cancerous bony lesions, a history of radiation to the bone, hypercalcemia, or a metabolic bone disease other than osteoporosis.[68] Although osteosarcoma has been described in rodents treated with teriparatide, no clear increase in the rate of cases has been reported in humans associated with this therapy.

Other Prescription Treatments

Other available osteoporosis treatments include selective estrogen receptor modulators (SERMs) (raloxifene [Evista]) and calcitonin (Fortical, Miacalcin). These agents have some benefit in the reduction of vertebral fracture risk, but no significant risk reduction at nonvertebral sites.[69,70]

SUMMARY

Osteoporosis is a common disorder seen daily by many orthopedic surgeons. Current recommendations from agencies and oversight bodies in the United States[33,71,72] recommend that all women 65 years and older undergo screening for osteoporosis with a DXA scan. However, a DXA is not required to make the diagnosis of osteoporosis if the patient has a history of a nontraumatic fracture. The FRAX calculator tool can assist in determining an individual's 10-year absolute fracture risk. Preventive measures, including calcium and vitamin D supplementation as well as precautions regarding the risk of falls, are very important in the care of patients at risk of fracture. However, for patients with a heightened fracture risk, prescription antiosteoporosis treatment should be considered, several options for which are available at present. Each treatment has associated benefits and potential risks, and these should be weighed on an individual basis with each patient. Further research is needed to assist clinicians in making decisions about long-term treatment of patients at risk. Until such questions are answered with longer-term studies, duration of use of antiresorptive treatments should be determined based on each patient's fracture risk; for many patients such treatment may be of finite duration.

REFERENCES

1. NOF fast facts. Available at: http://www.nof.org/node/40. Accessed August 27, 2012.
2. Burge R, Dawson-Hughes B, Solomon DH, et al. Incidence and economic burden of osteoporosis-related fractures in the United States, 2005-2025. J Bone Miner Res 2007;22(3):465–75.
3. Gehlbach S, Saag KG, Adachi JD, et al. Previous fractures at multiple sites increase the risk for subsequent fractures: the Global Longitudinal Study of Osteoporosis in Women. J Bone Miner Res 2012; 27(3):645–53.
4. Kanis JA, Johnell O, Oden A, et al. FRAX and the assessment of fracture probability in men and women from the UK. Osteoporos Int 2008;19(4): 385–97.
5. Watts NB, Adler RA, Bilezikian JP, et al. Osteoporosis in men: an Endocrine Society clinical practice guideline. J Clin Endocrinol Metab 2012;97(6): 1802–22.
6. Ebeling PR. Clinical practice. Osteoporosis in men. N Engl J Med 2008;358(14):1474–82.
7. Center JR, Bliuc D, Nguyen TV, et al. Risk of subsequent fracture after low-trauma fracture in men and women. JAMA 2007;297(4):387–94.
8. Cuddihy MT, Gabriel SE, Crowson CS, et al. Forearm fractures as predictors of subsequent osteoporotic fractures. Osteoporos Int 1999;9(6):469–75.
9. Mackey DC, Lui LY, Cawthon PM, et al. High-trauma fractures and low bone mineral density in older women and men. JAMA 2007;298(20):2381–8.
10. Sanders KM, Pasco JA, Ugoni AM, et al. The exclusion of high trauma fractures may underestimate the prevalence of bone fragility fractures in the community: the Geelong Osteoporosis Study. J Bone Miner Res 1998;13(8):1337–42.
11. Karlsson MK, Hasserius R, Obrant KJ. Individuals who sustain nonosteoporotic fractures continue to

also sustain fragility fractures. Calcif Tissue Int 1993; 53(4):229–31.

12. Melton LJ 3rd, Atkinson EJ, O'Fallon WM, et al. Long-term fracture prediction by bone mineral assessed at different skeletal sites. J Bone Miner Res 1993;8(10):1227–33.

13. Hedlund R, Lindgren U. Trauma type, age, and gender as determinants of hip fracture. J Orthop Res 1987;5(2):242–6.

14. Marks R, Mason B, Horne A, et al. Hip fractures among the elderly: causes, consequences and control. Ageing Res Rev 2003;2(1):57–93.

15. Suzuki T, Kim H, Yoshida H, et al. Randomized controlled trial of exercise intervention for the prevention of falls in community-dwelling elderly Japanese women. J Bone Miner Metab 2004;22(6):602–11.

16. Stevens JA, Olson S. Reducing falls and resulting hip fractures among older women. MMWR Recomm Rep 2000;49(RR-2):3–12.

17. Kita K, Hujino K, Nasu T, et al. A simple protocol for preventing falls and fractures in elderly individuals with musculoskeletal disease. Osteoporos Int 2007; 18(5):611–9.

18. Walker M, Klentrou P, Chow R, et al. Longitudinal evaluation of supervised versus unsupervised exercise programs for the treatment of osteoporosis. Eur J Appl Physiol 2000;83(4–5):349–55.

19. Gregg EW, Cauley JA, Seeley DG, et al. Physical activity and osteoporotic fracture risk in older women. Study of Osteoporotic Fractures Research Group. Ann Intern Med 1998;129(2):81–8.

20. Fiatarone MA, O'Neill EF, Ryan ND, et al. Exercise training and nutritional supplementation for physical frailty in very elderly people. N Engl J Med 1994; 330(25):1769–75.

21. Province MA, Hadley EC, Hornbrook MC, et al. The effects of exercise on falls in elderly patients. A pre-planned meta-analysis of the FICSIT trials. Frailty and Injuries: Cooperative Studies of Intervention Techniques. JAMA 1995;273(17):1341–7.

22. Greenspan SL, Myers ER, Kiel DP, et al. Fall direction, bone mineral density, and function: risk factors for hip fracture in frail nursing home elderly. Am J Med 1998;104(6):539–45.

23. Laing AC, Robinovitch SN. Effect of soft shell hip protectors on pressure distribution to the hip during sideways falls. Osteoporos Int 2008;19(7):1067–75.

24. Parker MJ, Gillespie WJ, Gillespie LD. Hip protectors for preventing hip fractures in older people. Cochrane Database Syst Rev 2005;(3):CD001255.

25. Kiel DP, Magaziner J, Zimmerman S, et al. Efficacy of a hip protector to prevent hip fracture in nursing home residents: the HIP PRO randomized controlled trial. JAMA 2007;298(4):413–22.

26. Reid IR, Mason B, Horne A, et al. Randomized controlled trial of calcium in healthy older women. Am J Med 2006;119(9):777–85.

27. Prince RL, Devine A, Dhaliwal SS, et al. Effects of calcium supplementation on clinical fracture and bone structure: results of a 5-year, double-blind, placebo-controlled trial in elderly women. Arch Intern Med 2006;166(8):869–75.

28. Lyons RA, Johansen A, Brophy S, et al. Preventing fractures among older people living in institutional care: a pragmatic randomised double blind placebo controlled trial of vitamin D supplementation. Osteoporos Int 2007;18(6):811–8.

29. Grant AM, Avenell A, Campbell MK, et al. Oral vitamin D3 and calcium for secondary prevention of low-trauma fractures in elderly people (Randomised Evaluation of Calcium Or vitamin D, RECORD): a randomised placebo-controlled trial. Lancet 2005;365(9471):1621–8.

30. Chapuy MC, Arlot ME, Duboeuf F, et al. Vitamin D3 and calcium to prevent hip fractures in the elderly women. N Engl J Med 1992;327(23):1637–42.

31. Dawson-Hughes B, Harris SS, Krall EA, et al. Effect of calcium and vitamin D supplementation on bone density in men and women 65 years of age or older. N Engl J Med 1997;337(10):670–6.

32. Larsen ER, Mosekilde L, Foldspang A. Vitamin D and calcium supplementation prevents osteoporotic fractures in elderly community dwelling residents: a pragmatic population-based 3-year intervention study. J Bone Miner Res 2004;19(3): 370–8.

33. U.S. Preventive Services Task Force. Screening for osteoporosis: U.S. preventive services task force recommendation statement. Ann Intern Med 2011; 154(5):356–64.

34. Papadimitropoulos E, Wells G, Shea B, et al. Meta-analyses of therapies for postmenopausal osteoporosis. VIII: meta-analysis of the efficacy of vitamin D treatment in preventing osteoporosis in postmenopausal women. Endocr Rev 2002;23(4): 560–9.

35. Lips P, Graafmans WC, Ooms ME, et al. Vitamin D supplementation and fracture incidence in elderly persons. A randomized, placebo-controlled clinical trial. Ann Intern Med 1996;124(4):400–6.

36. Heikinheimo RJ, Inkovaara JA, Harju EJ, et al. Annual injection of vitamin D and fractures of aged bones. Calcif Tissue Int 1992;51(2):105–10.

37. Bischoff-Ferrari HA, Willett WC, Wong JB, et al. Fracture prevention with vitamin D supplementation: a meta-analysis of randomized controlled trials. JAMA 2005;293(18):2257–64.

38. Jackson RD, LaCroix AZ, Gass M, et al. Calcium plus vitamin D supplementation and the risk of fractures. N Engl J Med 2006;354(7):669–83.

39. Bischoff-Ferrari HA, Willett WC, Orav EJ, et al. A pooled analysis of vitamin D dose requirements for fracture prevention. N Engl J Med 2012;367(1): 40–9.

40. Flicker L, Mead K, MacInnis RJ, et al. Serum vitamin D and falls in older women in residential care in Australia. J Am Geriatr Soc 2003;51(11):1533–8.

41. Bischoff HA, Stahelin HB, Dick W, et al. Effects of vitamin D and calcium supplementation on falls: a randomized controlled trial. J Bone Miner Res 2003;18(2):343–51.

42. Harwood RH, Sahota O, Gaynor K, et al. A randomised, controlled comparison of different calcium and vitamin D supplementation regimens in elderly women after hip fracture: the Nottingham Neck of Femur (NONOF) Study. Age Ageing 2004; 33(1):45–51.

43. Broe KE, Chen TC, Weinberg J, et al. A higher dose of vitamin D reduces the risk of falls in nursing home residents: a randomized, multiple-dose study. J Am Geriatr Soc 2007;55(2):234–9.

44. Bischoff-Ferrari HA, Orav EJ, Dawson-Hughes B. Effect of cholecalciferol plus calcium on falling in ambulatory older men and women: a 3-year randomized controlled trial. Arch Intern Med 2006;166(4): 424–30.

45. Flicker L, MacInnis RJ, Stein MS, et al. Should older people in residential care receive vitamin D to prevent falls? Results of a randomized trial. J Am Geriatr Soc 2005;53(11):1881–8.

46. Moyer VA. Prevention of falls in community-dwelling older adults: U.S. Preventive Services Task Force Recommendation Statement. Ann Intern Med 2012; 157(3):197–204.

47. Holick MF. Vitamin D deficiency. N Engl J Med 2007; 357(3):266–81.

48. Chapuy MC, Preziosi P, Maamer M, et al. Prevalence of vitamin D insufficiency in an adult normal population. Osteoporos Int 1997;7(5):439–43.

49. Holick MF, Siris ES, Binkley N, et al. Prevalence of Vitamin D inadequacy among postmenopausal North American women receiving osteoporosis therapy. J Clin Endocrinol Metab 2005;90(6):3215–24.

50. Gertner JM, Domenech M. 25-Hydroxyvitamin D levels in patients treated with high-dosage ergo- and cholecalciferol. J Clin Pathol 1977;30(2):144–50.

51. Vieth R. Vitamin D supplementation, 25-hydroxyvitamin D concentrations, and safety. Am J Clin Nutr 1999;69(5):842–56.

52. Ross AC, Manson JE, Abrams SA, et al. The 2011 report on dietary reference intakes for calcium and vitamin D from the Institute of Medicine: what clinicians need to know. J Clin Endocrinol Metab 2011; 96(1):53–8.

53. Holick MF, Binkley NC, Bischoff-Ferrari HA, et al. Evaluation, treatment, and prevention of vitamin D deficiency: an Endocrine Society clinical practice guideline. J Clin Endocrinol Metab 2011;96(7): 1911–30.

54. Wang L, Manson JE, Sesso HD. Calcium intake and risk of cardiovascular disease: a review of prospective studies and randomized clinical trials. Am J Cardiovasc Drugs 2012;12(2):105–16.

55. Bolland MJ, Grey A, Avenell A, et al. Calcium supplements with or without vitamin D and risk of cardiovascular events: reanalysis of the Women's Health Initiative limited access dataset and meta-analysis. BMJ 2011;342:d2040.

56. Bolland MJ, Avenell A, Baron JA, et al. Effect of calcium supplements on risk of myocardial infarction and cardiovascular events: meta-analysis. BMJ 2010;341:c3691.

57. Bolland MJ, Barber PA, Doughty RN, et al. Vascular events in healthy older women receiving calcium supplementation: randomised controlled trial. BMJ 2008;336(7638):262–6.

58. Paik J, Curhan G, Rexrode K, et al. A prospective study of calcium supplement intake and risk of cardiovascular disease in women. American Society for Bone and Mineral Research annual meeting. Abstract 1135. Minneapolis (MN), October 12–15, 2012.

59. Lyles KW, Colon-Emeric CS, Magaziner JS, et al. Zoledronic acid and clinical fractures and mortality after hip fracture. N Engl J Med 2007;357(18): 1799–809.

60. Liberman UA, Weiss SR, Broll J, et al. Effect of oral alendronate on bone mineral density and the incidence of fractures in postmenopausal osteoporosis. The Alendronate Phase III Osteoporosis Treatment Study Group. N Engl J Med 1995;333(22): 1437–43.

61. Pols HA, Felsenberg D, Hanley DA, et al. Multinational, placebo-controlled, randomized trial of the effects of alendronate on bone density and fracture risk in postmenopausal women with low bone mass: results of the FOSIT study. Fosamax International Trial Study Group. Osteoporos Int 1999;9(5):461–8.

62. Harris ST, Watts NB, Genant HK, et al. Effects of risedronate treatment on vertebral and nonvertebral fractures in women with postmenopausal osteoporosis: a randomized controlled trial. Vertebral Efficacy With Risedronate Therapy (VERT) Study Group. JAMA 1999;282(14):1344–52.

63. Delmas PD, Recker RR, Chesnut CH, et al. Daily and intermittent oral ibandronate normalize bone turnover and provide significant reduction in vertebral fracture risk: results from the BONE study. Osteoporos Int 2004;15(10):792–8.

64. Black DM, Delmas PD, Eastell R, et al. Once-yearly zoledronic acid for treatment of postmenopausal osteoporosis. N Engl J Med 2007;356(18): 1809–22.

65. Bekker PJ, Holloway DL, Rasmussen AS, et al. A single-dose placebo-controlled study of AMG 162, a fully human monoclonal antibody to RANKL, in postmenopausal women. 2004. J Bone Miner Res 2005;20(12):2275–82.

66. Whitaker M, Guo J, Kehoe T, et al. Bisphosphonates for osteoporosis—where do we go from here? N Engl J Med 2012;366(22):2048–51.

67. Black DM, Bauer DC, Schwartz AV, et al. Continuing bisphosphonate treatment for osteoporosis–for whom and for how long? N Engl J Med 2012; 366(22):2051–3.

68. Deal C, Gideon J. Recombinant human PTH 1-34 (Forteo): an anabolic drug for osteoporosis. Cleve Clin J Med 2003;70(7):585–6, 589–90, 592–4. passim.

69. Miacalcin® Nasal spray [package insert]. East Hanover (NJ): Novartis Pharmaceuticals Corporation. 2003.

70. Evista (raloxifene) [package insert]. Indianapolis (IN): Eli Lilly and Company. 2007.

71. Bone health and osteoporosis: a report of the Surgeon General. 2004. Available at: http://www.surgeongeneral.gov/library/reports/bonehealth/chapter_8.html#Step1 IdentifyAtRiskIndividualsWhoRequireFurtherEvaluation. Accessed February 22, 2011.

72. Clinician's guide to prevention and treatment of osteoporosis. 2010. Available at: http://www.nof.org/files/nof/public/content/file/344/upload/159.pdf. Accessed December 4, 2012

73. Alendronate package insert. Available at: http://www.merck.com/product/usa/pi_circulars/f/fosamax/fosamax_pi.pdf. Accessed August 27, 2012.

74. Wells GA, Cranney A, Peterson J, et al. Alendronate for the primary and secondary prevention of osteoporotic fractures in postmenopausal women. Cochrane Database Syst Rev 2008;(1):CD001155.

75. Ibandronate package insert. Available at: http://www.accessdata.fda.gov/drugsatfda_docs/label/2005/021455s001lbl.pdf. Accessed August 27, 2012.

76. Chesnut IC, Skag A, Christiansen C, et al. Effects of oral ibandronate administered daily or intermittently on fracture risk in postmenopausal osteoporosis. J Bone Miner Res 2004;19(8):1241–9.

77. Risedronate Package Insert. Available at: http://www.actonel.com/global/prescribing_information.pdf. Accessed August 27, 2012.

78. Wells G, Cranney A, Peterson J, et al. Risedronate for the primary and secondary prevention of osteoporotic fractures in postmenopausal women. Cochrane Database Syst Rev 2008;(1):CD004523.

79. Reclast package insert. Available at: http://www.pharma.us.novartis.com/product/pi/pdf/reclast.pdf. Accessed August 27, 2012.

80. Prolia package insert. Available at: http://pi.amgen.com/united_states/prolia/prolia_pi.pdf. Accessed August 27, 2012.

81. Cummings SR, San Martin J, McClung MR, et al. Denosumab for prevention of fractures in postmenopausal women with osteoporosis. N Engl J Med 2009;361(8):756–65.

82. Miacalcin package insert. Available at: http://www.pharma.us.novartis.com/product/pi/pdf/miacalcin_nasal.pdf. Accessed August 27, 2012.

83. Overgaard K, Hansen MA, Jensen SB, et al. Effect of salcatonin given intranasally on bone mass and fracture rates in established osteoporosis: a dose-response study. BMJ 1992;305(6853):556–61.

84. Evista package insert. Available at: http://pi.lilly.com/us/evista-pi.pdf. Accessed August 27, 2012.

85. Ettinger B, Black DM, Mitlak BH, et al. Reduction of vertebral fracture risk in postmenopausal women with osteoporosistreated with raloxifene: results from a 3-year randomized clinical trial. Multiple Outcomes of Raloxifene Evaluation (MORE) Investigators. JAMA 1999;282(7):637–45.

86. Forteo package insert. Available at: http://pi.lilly.com/us/forteo-pi.pdf. Accessed August 27, 2012.

87. Neer RM, Arnaud CD, Zanchetta JR, et al. Effect of parathyroid hormone (1-34) on fractures and bone mineral density in postmenopausal women with osteoporosis. N Engl J Med 2001;344(19):1434–41.

Bisphosphonate Therapy and Atypical Fractures

Anas Saleh, MD[a], Vishal V. Hegde, BA[b],
Anish G. Potty, MD[a], Joseph M. Lane, MD[a],*

KEYWORDS

- Bisphosphonate therapy • Atypical fractures • Osteoporosis • Atypical femoral fractures

KEY POINTS

- Bisphosphonate therapy is safe and effective for the management of osteoporosis when used for the duration measured in the original trials (<5 years).
- Atypical fractures constitute a rare subset of subtrochanteric and femoral shaft fractures.
- Careful identification and evaluation of these fractures demonstrated an association with prolonged bisphosphonate therapy (>5 years).
- Prolonged bisphosphonate therapy may contribute to atypical fractures by oversuppressing bone remodeling, leading to alterations in bone mineral and organic properties.
- Once atypical fractures are identified, bisphosphonates must be stopped and teriparatide therapy should be considered to enhance fracture healing.

INTRODUCTION

Bisphosphonates are a mainstay of therapy for osteoporosis. Several studies have documented their efficacy in preventing both vertebral and nonvertebral fractures.[1–4] With its continued success in improving bone mineral density and reducing the incidence of some fractures associated with low bone mass, longer-term data regarding bisphosphonate use have become available. Although described before the Food and Drug Administration's (FDA) approval and widespread clinical use of bisphosphonates, an uncommon variant of subtrochanteric and femoral shaft fractures thought to be associated with prolonged bisphosphonate therapy has captured the attention of the osteoporosis community. These so-called atypical femoral fractures occur after minimal trauma and have a distinct configuration and radiographic appearance compared with typical osteoporotic fractures. Although there is no evidence to suggest a cause-and-effect relationship, several studies have established an association between long-term bisphosphonate therapy and atypical femoral fractures.[5,6] Yet, several other clinical studies have provided data to counter this association.[7–9] This article highlights the reported incidence of atypical femoral fractures and their association with prolonged bisphosphonate therapy. The potential pathogenic mechanisms are discussed to identify gaps in our knowledge that warrant further research. A management approach is also provided to help guide orthopedic surgeons in the treatment of these fractures.

THE EMERGENCE OF ATYPICAL FEMORAL FRACTURES

When the early reports raised concerns regarding the possible link between bisphosphonate therapy

Disclosures: JML consults for Amgen, BioMimetic Therapeutics Inc, Bone Therapeutics SA, CollPlant, Ltd, Graftys SA, and Zimmer and serves on the Speakers Bureau for Eli Lilly, Novartis, and Warner Chilcott. All other authors state that they have no conflicts of interest.

[a] Department of Orthopaedic Surgery, Hospital for Special Surgery, 535 East 70th street, New York, NY 10021, USA; [b] Weill Cornell Medical College, Cornell University, 445 East 69th street, New York, NY 10021, USA
* Corresponding author. Metabolic Bone Disease Service, Department of Orthopaedic Surgery, Hospital for Special Surgery, New York, NY 10021.
E-mail address: Lanej@hss.edu

Orthop Clin N Am 44 (2013) 137–151
http://dx.doi.org/10.1016/j.ocl.2013.01.001
0030-5898/13/$ – see front matter © 2013 Published by Elsevier Inc.

and atypical fractures, most case series described a low-energy subtrochanteric or femoral shaft fracture in patients on prolonged bisphosphonate therapy. On further histologic examination, these patients seemed to have severely suppressed bone turnover.[10,11] Subsequent retrospective reports identified an atypical radiographic pattern as a simple transverse or oblique, noncomminuted fracture configuration with a medial spike, and cortical thickening (**Fig. 1**E).[12,13] This pattern was found to be particularly associated with prolonged bisphosphonate use.[14] Furthermore, prodromal pain and a periosteal stress reaction preceding the complete fracture were reported; these findings were consistent with stress fracture propagation (see **Fig. 1**A–D).[11,15]

The American Society for Bone and Mineral Research (ASBMR) soon recognized the occurrence of atypical femoral fractures, often in the setting of bisphosphonate use, and sought to provide diagnostic criteria to facilitate the proper identification of such fractures. In 2010, a task force of multidisciplinary experts reviewed available clinical evidence and defined major and minor features of atypical fractures (**Table 1**).[16] According to this definition, for a fracture to be considered atypical, all major features must be present, whereas minor features are not required to make the diagnosis. However, this definition remains subject to change and revision as more data become available.

EPIDEMIOLOGY: REASONS FOR CONTROVERSY

Atypical femoral fractures and their association with bisphosphonate therapy continue to be a controversial subject. Low level of evidence, controversial defining features, the use of diagnostic codes rather than radiographic adjudication, inadequate power, and short duration of the original trials are some of the limitations that impede accurate reporting and identification of a true association between bisphosphonate therapy and atypical fractures. In this section of the article, the authors discuss the epidemiologic evidence from larger cohort studies and clinical trials in light of these limitations.

Low Level of Evidence

The available evidence regarding the incidence of atypical femoral fractures and their association with prolonged bisphosphonate therapy comes from several case-control studies and several large retrospective cohort studies using national registries.[16–18] Therefore, the available level of evidence of this particular type of fracture is largely limited to levels III and IV.[19] Although prospective studies are required to properly answer the question of incidence and association, the rarity of these fractures calls for a large multicenter effort to achieve sufficient statistical power.

A Debatable Definition: What is Major and What is Minor?

Although the definition set forth by the ASBMR task force does not require minor features for the diagnosis of atypical femoral fractures, this definition may have to be revised in light of recent work by Feldstein and colleagues.[20] This study reviewed both electronic medical records and radiographs of women older than 50 years and men older than 65 years between 1996 and 2009 at Kaiser Permanente Northwest to describe incidence rates and characteristics of atypical fractures. By using the ASBMR major and minor radiographic criteria, they subdivided atypical femoral fractures into those with major features only and those with both major and minor features (localized periosteal reaction of the lateral cortex [beaking] and generalized cortical thickness). According to this definition, the incidence of typical femoral fractures and atypical fractures with major features only remained flat over the study period (cumulative incidence: 18.2 per 100 000 person-years and 5.9 per 100 000 person-years, respectively), whereas the proportion of atypical fractures with both major and minor features increased over time (**Fig. 2**). Moreover, patients with atypical fractures with only major features had a lower frequency of prolonged bisphosphonate use (2%) and prodromal pain (0%) compared with those with both major and minor features (29% and 27%, respectively). This study serves to create a more precise case definition of atypical femoral fractures and suggests that future research should evaluate fractures with minor features (localized periosteal reaction and cortical thickness) separately. Making this distinction not only affects incidence rates and association with bisphosphonate therapy but also advances our understanding of these fractures and has pathophysiological implications.

According to the ASBMR case definition, the minor criteria consist of either a localized periosteal reaction on the lateral cortex (beaking) or a generalized increase in cortical thickness of the diaphysis (see **Fig. 1**).[16] Because a higher proportion of patients with minor features had a history of bisphosphonate use, the study by Feldstein and colleagues revisits the association between bisphosphonate therapy and cortical thickening. However, it is important to make

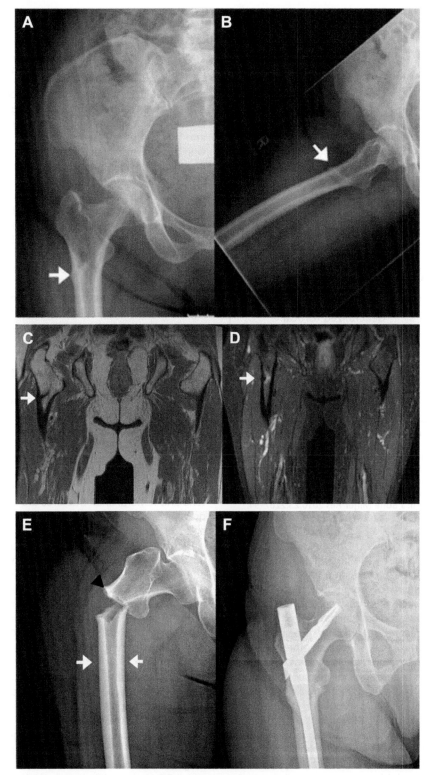

Fig. 1. A 66-year-old woman presented with thigh discomfort for 2 months without history of trauma. She had been on alendronate for 4 years. An anteroposterior femur radiograph revealed an incomplete atypical fracture with a periosteal reaction of the lateral cortex in the subtrochanteric area (*A, arrow*), and a lateral view showed a clear radiolucent fracture line (*B, arrow*); findings indicate a stress fracture. Magnetic resonance imaging showed the fracture line extending from the lateral to medial cortex on coronal T1-weighted image (*C, arrow*), with evident bone marrow edema on the short-tau inversion-recovery image (*D, arrow*). Two weeks after her initial presentation, the patient fell from standing height and sustained an atypical subtrochanteric femoral fracture. An anteroposterior radiograph of the right femur showed a transverse subtrochanteric fracture, with a localized periosteal thickening beaking (*black arrowhead*) and generalized cortical thickening (*white arrows*) (*E*). Four months after intramedullary nail fixation, the patient reported resolution of pain and improved function, with complete radiographic healing (*F*).

Table 1
ASBMR provisional case definition of atypical femoral fractures

Major features	Location: anywhere distal to lesser trochanter down to the supracondylar flare
	Configuration: transverse or short oblique
	No trauma or low-energy trauma
	Noncomminuted
	Medial spike in complete fracture
	Incomplete fracture only in the lateral cortex
Minor features	Localized periosteal reaction in the lateral cortex beaking
	Generalized cortical thickening
	Prodromal thigh pain or discomfort
	Bilaterality
	Delayed healing
	Bisphosphonate or glucocorticoid use

All major features are required to designate a fracture atypical; minor features are not required but have been associated with atypical fractures.

Data from Shane E, Burr D, Ebeling PR, et al. Atypical subtrochanteric and diaphyseal femoral fractures: report of a task force of the American Society for Bone and Mineral Research. J Bone Miner Res 2010;25:2267–94.

the distinction between the localized cortical thickening caused by the periosteal reaction and generalized cortical thickening. In a retrospective radiological study of complete subtrochanteric and femoral shaft fractures, cortical stress reaction (localized cortical thickness or beaking) had the highest odds ratio for predicting prior bisphosphonate use among other atypical features.[21] On the other hand, generalized cortical thickening, as assessed from the subtrochanteric region using dual-energy x-ray absorptiometry, did not seem to be common in long-term bisphosphonate users.[22] Although it remains to be determined whether generalized cortical thickening serves as a marker for propensity to sustain atypical fractures, a recent large population-based cohort of bisphosphonate-naïve women showed that subtrochanteric cortical thickening does not increase the risk of subtrochanteric, femoral shaft, or typical hip fractures.[23] Collectively, these findings emphasize our incomplete understanding of these features and the need for a revised definition of atypical femoral fractures.

The Use of Diagnostic Codes in Large National Registries Without Radiographic Adjudication

Large health databases provide advantages in power, real-world validity, and longer follow-up durations over clinical trials for assessing the harms and benefits of preventive medications. However, with regard to atypical femoral fractures, large health databases are not without limitations. Registers use diagnostic codes to capture patients with subtrochanteric and femoral shaft fractures. It is important to realize that not every subtrochanteric fracture is an atypical fracture. Typical subtrochanteric and femoral shaft fractures usually occur with high-energy trauma, are comminuted, and have a spiral configuration as opposed to the atypical fractures defined by the ASBMR.[24,25] As of yet, no diagnostic code has been assigned to atypical fractures; therefore, registers using diagnostic codes cannot distinguish between an atypical subtrochanteric fracture and a typical, osteoporotic subtrochanteric fracture. Previous studies that examined individual radiographs of patients with subtrochanteric or femoral shaft fractures reported that 2.3% to 34.0% of atypical fractures were miscoded by International Classification of Diseases codes.[20,26] Furthermore, information on trauma mechanism (low-energy trauma being one of the major features of atypical fractures) may be missing or uncertain. Therefore, studies that individually examined radiographs of patients with subtrochanteric and femoral shaft fractures are more valid for drawing conclusions regarding trends, risk factors, and associations.

With careful radiographic identification in large databases, atypical fractures seem to be uncommon (**Table 2**). In the Kaiser Permanente Northwest study, as described earlier, the rate of atypical femoral fractures with major and minor criteria seem to have increased from no events in the period between 1996 and 1999 to 5 per 100 0000 patient-years in 2009, along with a decline in classical hip fractures (see **Fig. 2**).[20] In another study using the National Swedish Patients Register, probably the largest database of patients who sustained femoral fractures, Schilcher and colleagues[5] performed a nationwide cohort analysis in 12 777 women aged 55 years and older who sustained a femoral fracture in Sweden in 2008. They reviewed radiographs of 1234 subtrochanteric fractures of which 59 were identified as atypical, with an overall rate of 4 per 100 000 person-years and 55 per 100 000 among bisphosphonate users. Giusti and colleagues[26] also reviewed the radiographs of 906 consecutive patients admitted into a single center with femoral fractures and showed a low prevalence of atypical fractures (1.1% of all femoral

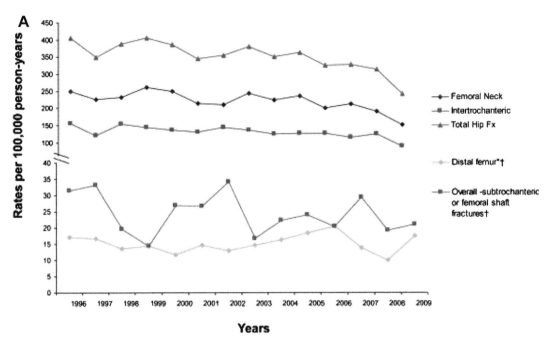

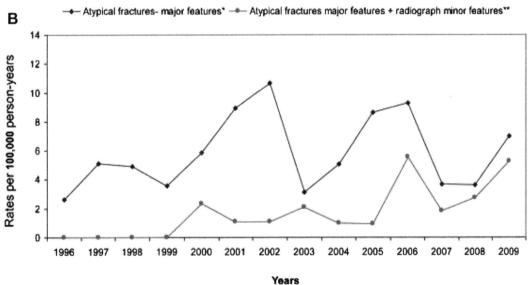

Fig. 2. (*A*) Incidence rates of femoral neck, intertrochanteric, and distal one-third femur fractures, and overall subtotal hip fractures. [a] Distal femur means distal to condylar flare. [b] Rates are graphed on a different scale than the hip fractures. (*B*) Incidence rates of subtrochanteric or femoral shaft fracture subtypes based on radiograph review. Major and minor features of ASBMR are summarized in **Table 1**. (*Reprinted from* Feldstein A, Black D, Perrin N, et al. Incidence and demography of femur fractures with and without atypical features. J Bone Miner Res 2012;27:977–86; This material is reproduced with permission of John Wiley & Sons, Inc.)

fractures and 10.4% of all subtrochanteric or femoral shaft fractures).

In large databases without radiographic adjudication, it remains possible to examine whether there is a shift from classical hip fractures to other femur fractures since the introduction of bisphosphonates in 1996. Wang and Bhattacharyya[27] analyzed national trends in hip and femur fractures between 1996 and 2007 by retrospectively using the National Inpatient Sample, Medical Expenditure Panel Surgery, and National Hospital Discharge Survey (NHDS) databases. The results showed that during

Table 2
The incidence of atypical femoral fractures as determined by 3 large observational studies with radiograph adjudication

Study	Data Source	Number of Fractures	Prevalence of Atypical Fractures
Feldstein et al,[20] 2012	Kaiser Permanente Northwest	5034 Femoral fractures 122 ST/FS 75 Atypical	5.9 per 100 000 person-years
Schilcher et al,[5] 2011	National Swedish Patient Register	12 777 Femoral fractures 263 ST/FS 59 Atypical	4 per 100 000 person-years
Giusti et al,[26] 2011	Single center in the Netherlands	906 Femoral fractures 53 ST/FS 10 Atypical	1.1% of all femoral fractures and 10.4% of ST/FS fractures

Abbreviation: ST/FS, subtrochanteric/femoral shaft.

this period, rates for typical fractures decreased by 32% in women and 20% in men, whereas the overall trends in subtrochanteric fractures remained unchanged in men and increased by 20% in women. Another study by Nieves and colleagues[28] using the NHDS also analyzed the trends for distinct subtypes of femoral fractures over a similar time period (1996–2006) and found a significant decline in incidence rates of hip fractures but not in subtrochanteric fractures, which remained stable at 20 per 100 000 person-years in women. Collectively, studies with and without radiograph adjudication clearly show that atypical femoral fractures constitute a small subset of subtrochanteric and femoral shaft fractures, which in turn account for only 3% to 5% of all femoral fractures.[28]

Several cohort and matched case-control studies were conducted to identify the risk of developing atypical femoral fractures in bisphosphonate users (**Table 3**). Again, most of these studies did not have radiograph adjudication to identify atypical fractures as such. Studies relying on large databases without reviewing radiographs have largely failed to demonstrate an increased risk of atypical fractures in bisphosphonate users.[7,9,29,30] Three studies used the Danish National Hospital Discharge database. The first study did not find a greater frequency of these fractures in bisphosphonate users[7]; the second one from the same group did demonstrate an increased risk, but not a dose-response relationship[29]; and the third study concluded that the risk of fracture was already present before the drugs were started and there was no dose-response relationship present.[30] However, one large Canadian, population-based, nested case-control study used data from the Ontario Public Drug Program database and showed that the risk of atypical fractures only increased in those who received bisphosphonates for longer than

5 years.[6] As mentioned earlier, the biggest study to specifically look at the risk of atypical fractures using radiographs was by Schilcher and colleagues[5]; it demonstrated an increased relative risk (RR) in the cohort analysis (RR 47.3; 95% confidence interval [CI], 25.6–87.3) and an increased odds ratio (OR) of 33.3 (95% CI, 14.3–77.8). Even more interesting, the investigators were able to demonstrate a 70% reduction in the RR per year after drug withdrawal (OR 0.28; 95% CI, 0.21–0.38). The fact that radiographs were individually examined in this study grants more validity to the results over other registry-based studies.

The Inherent Limitations of the Original Trials

Randomized clinical trials are efficacy trials by design and are not powered to look at adverse effects, especially rare adverse effects, such as atypical fractures. In addition to having too few participants, follow-up times are often short; and in some populations, comorbidities and additional drug interactions may not be adequately represented in earlier phases of clinical testing. The true safety profile of any medication is really only understood after the medication has been on the market for a sufficiently long period of time and has been used by a large number of patients. This point is especially true in the case of atypical fractures because the pathogenesis involves time-dependent processes (see pathogenesis section later) rather than a dose-dependent adverse effect. Therefore, it was certainly difficult to anticipate a potential long-term complication when most phase trials were conducted for shorter durations.

Black and colleagues[8] performed secondary analyses using the results of 3 large randomized controlled trials: the Fracture Intervention Trial (FIT), the FIT Long-Term Extension (FLEX) trial,

Table 3
The risk of subtrochanteric and femoral shaft fractures in bisphosphonate users from large observational studies

Study	Data Source	Risk of ST/FS in Bisphosphonate Users	Conclusions
Abrahamsen et al,[7] 2009	Danish National Hospital Discharge database	HR = 1.46 (95% CI, 0.91–2.35)	ST/FS fractures share the epidemiology and treatment response of classical hip fractures and are best classified as osteoporotic fractures.
Abrahamsen et al,[29] 2010		HR = 2.66 (95% CI, 2.35–3.02)	• BP users are at a higher risk of hip or ST/FS fractures. • Large cumulative dose of BP was not associated with a greater absolute risk.
Vestergaard et al,[30] 2011		HR = 2.41 (95% CI, 1.78–3.27)	• There was an increased risk of ST/FS fractures, but patients had an increased risk before initiation of therapy. • There was no dose-response relationship.
Black et al,[8] 2010	Post hoc analysis of 3 randomized clinical trials	• FIT HR = 1.03 (95% CI, 0.06–16.46) • FLEX HR = 1.33 (95% CI, 0.12–14.67) • HORIZON HR = 1.50 (95% CI, 0.25–9.00)	There was no significant increase in risk, but the study was underpowered for a definitive diagnosis.
Kim et al,[9] 2011	Medicare beneficiaries in Pennsylvania and New Jersey	HR = 1.03 (95% CI, 0.70–1.52) compared with raloxifene/calcitonin	• The risk of atypical fractures is no greater with BP than is the case with weaker antiresorptives. • The study has little precision beyond 5 y.
Park-Wyllie et al,[6] 2011	Ontario Public Drug Program database	OR = 2.74 (95% CI, 1.25–6.05) >5 y of BP therapy	Treatment with BP for more than 5-y increased the risk of ST/FS fracture.
Schilcher et al,[5] 2011	National Swedish Patient Register	OR = 33.3 (95% CI, 14.3–77.8) for atypical fractures	• Atypical femoral fractures absolute risk is 5 per 10 000 person-years. • Risk diminished by 70% per year since the last use.

Abbreviations: BP, bisphosphonates; CI, confidence interval; FIT, Fracture Intervention Trial; FLEX, FIT Long-Term Extension trial; HORIZON, Health Outcomes and Reduced Incidence with Zoledronic Acid Once Yearly Pivotal Fracture Trial; HR, hazard ratio; OR, odds ratio; ST/FS, subtrochanteric/femoral shaft.

and the Health Outcomes and Reduced Incidence with Zoledronic Acid Once Yearly Pivotal Fracture Trial (HORIZON-PFT). The investigators showed that the relative hazard was not significant; but the 95% confidence intervals were wide, and original radiographs were generally unavailable at the time of the analysis. Furthermore, the 2 placebo-controlled trials (FIT and HORIZON-PFT) lasted only 3.0 to 4.5 years and, thus, could not assess whether the risk of fracture increased with treatment duration. Even in the FLEX trial, which included women who were treated up to 10 years, only 186 patients received more than 8 years of treatment, making the study strongly underpowered.

The lack of long-term exposure is a major problem when examining long-term outcomes, such as atypical fractures. Studies with access to a substantial number of femur radiographs from fracture patients have been limited by short-term drug history data. For example, although the study by Schilcher and colleagues[5] from Sweden used radiograph adjudication, it was constrained by having access to less than 3 years of medication history. What makes this more troublesome is that patients on bisphosphonates often have substantial treatment gaps and varying compliance rates, so that what would seem to be a bisphosphonate-naïve patient could be in fact a patient who had used bisphosphonate for many years but done so at a time when prescriptions were not yet captured.

It is clear that atypical femoral fractures are not common. An association with bisphosphonate therapy seems to exist based on studies that identified those fractures radiographically.[5,18] Large observation studies had to rely on diagnosis codes, resulting in incidence rates that are too high and odds ratios that are too low because they include fractures that may not be atypical. Yet the fact that many patients with skeletal malignancies receiving massive doses of bisphosphonate never develop these fractures,[31] and that some patients with atypical fractures have not used bisphosphonates, adds to the controversy. Longer-term drug exposure data linked to radiographs are required to elucidate an accurate association and optimal duration of bisphosphonate therapy.

PATHOGENESIS

Nitrogen-containing bisphosphonates (alendronate, ibandronate, risedronate, pamidronate, and zoledronic acid) act by inhibiting farnesyl pyrophosphate synthetase, a key enzyme in the production of cholesterol, leading to cellular apoptosis.[32,33] Bisphosphonates specifically target osteoclast-mediated bone resorption by virtue of their high affinity to bone. They are retained in bone until taken up by osteoclasts during bone resorption, leading to osteoclast apoptosis and suppression of bone turnover. The suppression of bone turnover provides the rationale for most pharmacologic interventions used for patients with postmenopausal osteoporosis. These antiresorptive medications improve the structural biomechanical properties of bone by increasing bone mass while maintaining bone microarchitecture, thus significantly reducing fracture risk.

Despite the beneficial effects of bone turnover suppression on bone strength and fracture risk, severe suppression of bone turnover is thought to play a major role in the development of atypical femoral fractures. Because bisphosphonates preferentially accumulate in areas of high osteogenic activity, such as sites of microfracture repair, their effects may be amplified locally, leading to alterations in microdamage physiology, mineralization and heterogeneity of mineral and organic matrix, and collagen cross-linking pattern.

Alterations in Microdamage Physiology

The accumulation of microdamage in bone is a normal physiologic event that occurs because of cyclic loading. In normal bone, microdamage initiates bone remodeling.[34] It is, thus, the suppression of bone remodeling caused by bisphosphonates that leads to the belief that an increase in microdamage accumulation is the natural consequence of bisphosphonate therapy. This theory out in studies that show that the magnitude of microdamage accumulation is inversely correlated to the level of bone turnover.[35–37] These increases in microdamage accumulation seem to occur most rapidly during the early phase of treatment.

Increased microdamage accumulation alone does not fully explain the role of prolonged bisphosphonate therapy in atypical fractures. Prolonged turnover suppression does not lead to ever-increasing levels of microdamage; instead, a plateau in damage accumulation is reached.[38] In an ovine model with the ability to undergo intracortical remodeling, it has been shown that bisphosphonates result in an increased number of microcracks; yet these microcracks were also shorter in length, making them less likely to negatively impact fracture risk.[39] Furthermore, a recent study in dogs demonstrated that the reduction in toughness apparent in bone after bisphosphonate treatment does not correspond to the accumulation of microdamage.[35] Regardless of the potential for increased microdamage accumulation in patients treated with bisphosphonate, a direct link between this microdamage accumulation and a decrease in bone toughness has yet to be established. It may be that this reduction in bone toughness caused by bisphosphonate therapy is mediated through other mechanisms. To date, there is still no substantive evidence linking bisphosphonates to microcrack formation in humans.

Increased Mineralization and Reduced Heterogeneity of Mineral and Organic Matrix

As a consequence of the reduction in bone turnover caused by bisphosphonates, the mineralization profile of bone is significantly altered. Bisphosphonates prolong the life of existing remodeling units and reduces the formation of new ones. This prolongation allows for a great percentage of bone remodeling units to become older and fully mineralized, leading to an increase in the homogeneity of mineralization.[40–42]

The increases in bone mineralization and mineralization homogeneity have important repercussions with regard to fracture risk. Although increased mineralization is positively correlated with increased strength and stiffness, it is negatively correlated with toughness.[36,37,43,44] Reductions in toughness are closely predicted by changes in mineralization and would contribute to increased brittleness of the bone and susceptibility to fracture.

The distribution of stress when bone is loaded is also impacted by the homogeneity of mineralization.[45] The variation in more heterogeneously comprised bone will produce areas of varying compliance and stiffness. Propagating cracks can be halted at an area because of this variance. Donnelly and colleagues[41] showed that the distribution of collagen maturity and crystal perfection in patients treated with bisphosphonate is significantly narrowed when compared with patients without bisphosphonate therapy. The increased homogeneity in the organic matrix, combined with the increased homogeneity of mineralization, may allow for further propagation of microcracks in bone and lead to a higher fracture risk in patients with prolonged bisphosphonate therapy.

Alterations to Collagen Cross-Linking

Collagen, which constitutes 90% of the organic matrix of bone, is cross-linked through both enzymatic and nonenzymatic processes.[46] The enzymatic process is mediated by lysyl and prolyl hydroxylases, resulting in trivalent collagen cross-links.[38] These cross-links yield a more stable collagen matrix and seem to be positively associated with stiffness and strength in bone.[47–49] Three years of bisphosphonate treatment did not affect the total amount of enzymatic cross-links in animal studies.[50]

Nonenzymatic cross-linking, on the other hand, occurs when reducing sugars interacts with free amino groups in collagen, resulting in advanced glycation end products (AGEs). Accumulation of AGEs is a result of delayed tissue turnover relative to the rate of formation because AGEs are removed when bone is remodeled. Thus, increased amounts of AGEs have been observed in aging bone and patients with diabetes.[51–53] Increased AGE concentration in bone has been shown to significantly reduce fracture resistance by increasing the brittleness of bone and decreasing bone toughness.[54–56]

Because bisphosphonates suppress bone turnover, thereby increasing mean tissue age, it is theorized that AGEs may also accumulate in bisphosphonate-treated bone. Multiple animal studies have shown that 1 to 3 years of treatment with a bisphosphonate results in an increase in AGEs in bone.[50,56,57] Unfortunately, there is no human data on the accumulation of AGEs in patients on long-term bisphosphonate therapy, so it is not clear to what extent AGEs would accumulate in these patients. It would be interesting to examine the incidence of atypical fractures in patients with diabetes with poor glycemic control because they would be expected to have accumulated more AGEs. The clinical study by Lo and colleagues[58] showed that patients with atypical fractures were less likely to have diabetes, but no information was available on their glycemic control.

Biomechanical Considerations

Femoral biomechanical differences may contribute to the risk of atypical fractures in susceptible patients. Atypical femoral fractures originate at the lateral cortex of the femur, from below the greater trochanter to approximately the midshaft; this is the area of highest tensile stress distribution in the femoral shaft.[59] Populations with bowed femurs are expected to have greater bending stress and be at greater risk for stress fracture initiation in the lateral cortex. The relationship between geometric factors, such as femoral bowing, and atypical femoral fractures has not been directly examined. However, Lo and colleagues[58] showed that patients with atypical femoral fractures are more likely to be Asian, a population known to have femoral bowing and different hip axis length.[60] Therefore, future research is warranted to further examine the relation between different mechanical parameters and atypical fractures.

PROLONGED BISPHOSPHONATE THERAPY: WHEN TO STOP

Because of a concern regarding oversuppression of bone turnover with prolonged bisphosphonate therapy and the risk of atypical fractures, the FDA performed a systematic review of long-term bisphosphonate efficacy by focusing on trials whereby bisphosphonates had been administered for at least 3 years (FLEX, HORIZON-PFT, and Vertebral Efficacy with Risedronate Trial-MultiNational).[61,62] Pooled data from these trials pertaining to patients who received continuous bisphosphonate treatment for 6 or more years results in fracture rates ranging from 9.3% to 10.6%, whereas the rate for patients switched to placebo is 8.0% to 8.8%. These data raise the question of whether continued bisphosphonate therapy imparts additional antifracture benefit relative to cessation of therapy after 5 years. It should be noted, however, that all fracture data in the FDA review are post hoc and are limited by statistical power, selection bias, and sample size.

To optimize the efficacy of bisphosphonates in reducing fractures, decisions to continue treatment must be individualized based on patients' risks and benefits. Black and colleagues[63] reevaluated their analyses of the extension trials and showed that stratifying patients according to their risk of fracture can help identify patients that would benefit the most from continuing therapy. Patients with low bone mineral density at the femoral neck (T score less than −2.5) or patients with an existing vertebral fracture seem to benefit the most from continued therapy, whereas patients with a femoral neck T score more than −2.0 have a low risk of vertebral fracture and are unlikely to benefit from continued treatment. These patients with a low risk of fracture can be placed on a drug holiday. Unfortunately, there is currently no data to guide clinicians in determining whether and when to resume treatment. The use of bisphosphonates with less binding affinity, such as risedronate, can be considered because their effects on bone turnover suppression can wear off sooner in the event of oversuppression.[64]

Bone turnover markers provide pharmacodynamic information on the level of suppression in response to bisphosphonate therapy and, as a result, are widely used for monitoring treatment. However, their clinical value for monitoring is limited by inadequate appreciation of the sources of variability, by limited data for comparison of treatments using the same markers, and by the lack of international reference standards.[65] The role of repeat assessment of bone mineral density, bone turnover markers, and other clinical indicators needs further evaluation.

MANAGEMENT OF ATYPICAL FRACTURES

The management of atypical fractures remains a challenge because of the lack of prospective studies evaluating different treatment protocols in these infrequent fractures. However, it is becoming clear that an approach combining both medical and surgical management is required to optimize outcomes in these patients.

Medical Management

1. Discontinue bisphosphonates

A large observational study from a health maintenance organization in California examined the occurrence of a contralateral atypical femur fracture after the index atypical fracture in patients who either continued or discontinued the use of bisphosphonates.[66] With radiographic adjudication, Dell and colleagues[66] identified 126 patients with atypical fractures who were on bisphosphonates. The study showed that the incidence of bilateral atypical femur fractures is 41% in patients who continued bisphosphonates for 3 or more years after the index atypical femur fracture versus 19% in patients who discontinued the drug. The risk of a contralateral atypical fracture is decreased by 53% if bisphosphonates were stopped after the index fracture. Similarly, the aforementioned study by Schilcher[5] demonstrated a 70% reduction in the RR of developing atypical fractures per year after bisphosphonate withdrawal.

2. Calcium and vitamin D supplementation

Calcium and vitamin D supplementation is one of the fundamentals of orthopedic practice, especially patients with fragility fractures. Vitamin D has been shown to be important for maintaining calcium homeostasis, improving muscle function, and preventing falls.[67,68] Furthermore, vitamin D and calcium supplementation has been proven to be effective at reducing the risk of all fractures by 12% to 26%.[69,70] Recommendations for optimal treatment should include daily calcium intake of 1000 to 1200 mg/d.[71] Although current recommendations from the Institute of Medicine (IOM) state that 400 to 800 IU/d of vitamin D3 is adequate, many experts and studies have shown these recommendations to be insufficient.[71,72] The minimum adult intake of vitamin D3 should be 1000 to 2000 IU/d,[73,74] along with regular monitoring of serum 25-hydroxyvitamin D and parathyroid hormone (PTH) levels. The goal is to maintain serum 25-hydroxyvitamin D levels more than 32 ng/mL[75,76] and prevent elevations in serum PTH.

3. Teriparatide (1–34 PTH)

Teriparatide, recombinant PTH 1–34 (PTH 1–34), must be considered in patients with atypical femoral fractures. It improves bone turnover and microarchitecture in patients on long-term alendronate treatment[77,78] and enhances fracture healing by increasing callus formation and mechanical strength.[79–82] Two clinical trials also showed that teriparatide shortened the time to healing in patients with osteoporotic fractures.[83,84] Although no randomized studies exist to examine the effect of teriparatide in atypical fractures specifically, these studies provide a solid argument for the use of teriparatide in these fractures to accelerate fracture healing and increase bone turnover.

Surgical Management of Complete Atypical Fractures

No studies have directly examined different surgical options for atypical fractures. Most surgeons, however, prefer the use of intramedullary nails because they offer biologic and biomechanical advantages (see **Fig. 1**F). Fractures treated by intramedullary nail heal by endochondral ossification, with an initial inflammatory response and formation of a cartilage callus. Bisphosphonates do not impair the initial phases of fracture healing or the development of a proliferative callus.[85,86] They only slow the remodeling phase, delaying the remodeling of the calcified cartilage callus to mature bone. Plates are inherently biomechanically inferior to nails because of their more lateral position (longer lever arm on the proximal fixation) and their non–load-sharing characteristics. They are also biologically inferior to nails because they require intramembranous healing, which is inhibited by bisphosphonates. Therefore, plate-screw constructs are not recommended for atypical femoral fractures. Plates, however, can be used when reduction is hard to achieve with nailing or when nailing is impractical because of thickened cortices.

Atypical femoral fractures take longer to heal after surgical fixation.[16] Weil and colleagues[87] demonstrated a poor surgical outcome for atypical fractures when 7 out of 16 fractures (53%) required

revision after the initial intramedullary nailing. In an effort to optimize bone healing and callus formation, preemptive autologous bone marrow grafting can be considered. Although no studies have examined the efficacy of this procedure in atypical fractures, autologous bone marrow grafting is a minimally invasive technique that proved to be successful in treating nonunions.[88–90] Furthermore, the use of osteoinductive materials, such as demineralized bone matrix and recombinant human morphogenic protein-2, should be explored in light of their ability to stimulate bone formation and fracture healing.[91,92]

Approach to Incomplete Atypical Fractures

Because of the high incidence of bilaterality in atypical femoral fractures,[16,18,58] it is recommended to evaluate the contralateral femur with plain radiographs. Lo and colleagues[58] showed that up to 40% of patients with atypical fractures had a contralateral stress or complete atypical fracture after the index fracture. By evaluating the contralateral femur, more incomplete atypical fractures are being identified, leaving the orthopedic surgeon with the dilemma of whether to perform surgical prophylaxis or conservative management on these incomplete fractures.

The management of incomplete atypical fractures depends on several factors, including

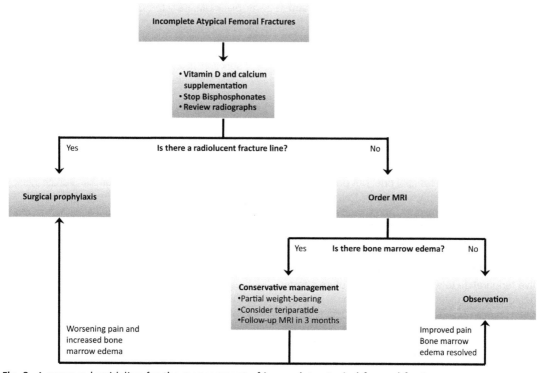

Fig. 3. A proposed guideline for the management of incomplete atypical femoral fractures.

symptoms, plain radiographs, and magnetic resonance imaging (MRI). Femur radiographs with cortical thickening and stress reaction should be carefully examined for the presence of a radiolucent fracture line across the lateral cortex (see **Fig. 1**A, B). The presence of this radiolucent fracture line seems to be a predictor of prognosis in such cases; fractures with a radiolucent fracture line have an increased propensity of progressing to complete fracture and failing conservative management.[93,94] Therefore, prophylactic fixation with an intramedullary nail is warranted in such patients to avoid progression to complete fracture. If patients are complaining of pain but without a discernable radiolucent fracture line on radiographs, MRI is required to look for bone marrow edema indicating an active stress fracture (see **Fig. 1**C, D). In these patients, a conservative approach can be undertaken, which involves partial weight-bearing with an assistive device, stopping the bisphosphonate, supplementing calcium and vitamin D, and starting teriparatide. Close follow-up with MRI is needed to monitor the resolution of bone marrow edema and prevent progression to complete fracture. Prophylactic fixation should be considered if there is persistent or worsening pain after conservative therapy (**Fig. 3**).

SUMMARY

Epidemiologic reports demonstrate that atypical femoral fractures are an uncommon subtype of subtrochanteric and femoral shaft fractures. Studies that correctly identified atypical femoral fractures by directly examining radiographs showed an increase risk of these fractures in long-term bisphosphonate users. However, this association does not prove causation. Most of the evidence for the pathogenesis for these fractures stems from animal studies with very limited applicability to human bone. Therefore, bisphosphonates remain safe and effective agents for the treatment of osteoporosis. The decision to terminate bisphosphonate after 5 years of therapy is still a controversial one, but patients with a low risk of fractures may not benefit from extended treatment periods. However, once an atypical fracture occurs, bisphosphonates must be stopped, and patients should receive daily calcium and vitamin D supplementation. The preferred method of fixation is by intramedullary nailing, with postoperative teriparatide to augment healing. Future efforts should focus on establishing a definitive set of diagnostic criteria and codes to accurately identify these fractures as well as explore histomorphometry and biomechanical properties of human femoral cortices. A multicenter effort is necessary to determine the best approach to manage these fractures.

REFERENCES

1. Black DM, Schwartz AV, Ensrud KE, et al. Effects of continuing or stopping alendronate after 5 years of treatment: the fracture intervention trial long-term extension (FLEX): a randomized trial. JAMA 2006; 296:2927–38.
2. Black DM, Delmas PD, Eastell R, et al. Once-yearly zoledronic acid for treatment of postmenopausal osteoporosis. N Engl J Med 2007;356:1809–22.
3. Chesnut CH III, Skag A, Christiansen C, et al. Effects of oral ibandronate administered daily or intermittently on fracture risk in postmenopausal osteoporosis. J Bone Miner Res 2004;19:1241–9.
4. Harris ST, Watts NB, Genant HK, et al. Effects of risedronate treatment on vertebral and nonvertebral fractures in women with postmenopausal osteoporosis: a randomized controlled trial. Vertebral efficacy with risedronate therapy (VERT) study group. JAMA 1999;282:1344–52.
5. Schilcher J, Michaelsson K, Aspenberg P. Bisphosphonate use and atypical fractures of the femoral shaft. N Engl J Med 2011;364:1728–37.
6. Park-Wyllie LY, Mamdani MM, Juurlink DN, et al. Bisphosphonate use and the risk of subtrochanteric or femoral shaft fractures in older women. JAMA 2011; 305:783–9.
7. Abrahamsen B, Eiken P, Eastell R. Subtrochanteric and diaphyseal femur fractures in patients treated with alendronate: a register-based national cohort study. J Bone Miner Res 2009;24:1095–102.
8. Black DM, Kelly MP, Genant HK, et al. Bisphosphonates and fractures of the subtrochanteric or diaphyseal femur. N Engl J Med 2010;362:1761–71.
9. Kim SY, Schneeweiss S, Katz JN, et al. Oral bisphosphonates and risk of subtrochanteric or diaphyseal femur fractures in a population-based cohort. J Bone Miner Res 2011;26:993–1001.
10. Odvina CV, Zerwekh JE, Rao DS, et al. Severely suppressed bone turnover: a potential complication of alendronate therapy. J Clin Endocrinol Metab 2005; 90:1294–301.
11. Goh SK, Yang KY, Koh JS, et al. Subtrochanteric insufficiency fractures in patients on alendronate therapy: a caution. J Bone Joint Surg Br 2007;89:349–53.
12. Lenart BA, Lorich DG, Lane JM. Atypical fractures of the femoral diaphysis in postmenopausal women taking alendronate. N Engl J Med 2008;358:1304–6.
13. Neviaser AS, Lane JM, Lenart BA, et al. Low-energy femoral shaft fractures associated with alendronate use. J Orthop Trauma 2008;22:346–50.
14. Lenart BA, Neviaser AS, Lyman S, et al. Association of low-energy femoral fractures with prolonged bisphosphonate use: a case control study. Osteoporos Int 2009;20:1353–62.
15. Kwek EB, Goh SK, Koh JS, et al. An emerging pattern of subtrochanteric stress fractures:

a long-term complication of alendronate therapy? Injury 2008;39:224–31.

16. Shane E, Burr D, Ebeling PR, et al. Atypical subtrochanteric and diaphyseal femoral fractures: report of a task force of the American Society for Bone and Mineral Research. J Bone Miner Res 2010;25:2267–94.

17. Rizzoli R, Akesson K, Bouxsein M, et al. Subtrochanteric fractures after long-term treatment with bisphosphonates: a European Society on Clinical and Economic Aspects of Osteoporosis and Osteoarthritis, and International Osteoporosis Foundation Working Group report. Osteoporos Int 2011;22:373–90.

18. Giusti A, Hamdy NA, Papapoulos SE. Atypical fractures of the femur and bisphosphonate therapy: a systematic review of case/case series studies. Bone 2010;47:169–80.

19. Wright JG, Swiontkowski M, Heckman JD. Levels of evidence. J Bone Joint Surg Br 2006;88:1264.

20. Feldstein A, Black D, Perrin N, et al. Incidence and demography of femur fractures with and without atypical features. J Bone Miner Res 2012;27:977–86.

21. Rosenberg ZS, La Rocca Vieira R, Chan SS, et al. Bisphosphonate-related complete atypical subtrochanteric femoral fractures: diagnostic utility of radiography. AJR Am J Roentgenol 2011;197:954–60.

22. Unnanuntana A, Ashfaq K, Ton QV, et al. The effect of long-term alendronate treatment on cortical thickness of the proximal femur. Clin Orthop Relat Res 2012;470:291–8.

23. Napoli N, Jin J, Peters K, et al. Are women with thicker cortices in the femoral shaft at higher risk of subtrochanteric/diaphyseal fractures? The study of osteoporotic fractures. J Clin Endocrinol Metab 2012. http://dx.doi.org/10.1210/jc.2011-3256.

24. Salminen S, Pihlajamaki H, Avikainen V, et al. Specific features associated with femoral shaft fractures caused by low-energy trauma. J Trauma 1997; 43:117–22.

25. Salminen ST, Pihlajamaki HK, Avikainen VJ, et al. Population based epidemiologic and morphologic study of femoral shaft fractures. Clin Orthop Relat Res 2000;372:241–9.

26. Giusti A, Hamdy NA, Dekkers OM, et al. Atypical fractures and bisphosphonate therapy: a cohort study of patients with femoral fracture with radiographic adjudication of fracture site and features. Bone 2011;48:966–71.

27. Wang Z, Bhattacharyya T. Trends in incidence of subtrochanteric fragility fractures and bisphosphonate use among the US elderly, 1996-2007. J Bone Miner Res 2011;26:553–60.

28. Nieves JW, Bilezikian JP, Lane JM, et al. Fragility fractures of the hip and femur: incidence and patient characteristics. Osteoporos Int 2010;21:399–408.

29. Abrahamsen B, Eiken P, Eastell R. Cumulative alendronate dose and the long-term absolute risk of subtrochanteric and diaphyseal femur fractures: a register-based national cohort analysis. J Clin Endocrinol Metab 2010;95:5258–65.

30. Vestergaard P, Schwartz F, Rejnmark L, et al. Risk of femoral shaft and subtrochanteric fractures among users of bisphosphonates and raloxifene. Osteoporos Int 2011;22:993–1001.

31. Puhaindran ME, Farooki A, Steensma MR, et al. Atypical subtrochanteric femoral fractures in patients with skeletal malignant involvement treated with intravenous bisphosphonates. J Bone Joint Surg Am 2011;93:1235–42.

32. Dunford JE, Thompson K, Coxon FP, et al. Structure-activity relationships for inhibition of farnesyl diphosphate synthase in vitro and inhibition of bone resorption in vivo by nitrogen-containing bisphosphonates. J Pharmacol Exp Ther 2001;296:235–42.

33. Luckman SP, Hughes DE, Coxon FP, et al. Nitrogen-containing bisphosphonates inhibit the mevalonate pathway and prevent post-translational prenylation of GTP-binding proteins, including Ras. J Bone Miner Res 1998;13:581–9.

34. Bentolila V, Boyce TM, Fyhrie DP, et al. Intracortical remodeling in adult rat long bones after fatigue loading. Bone 1998;23:275–81.

35. Allen MR, Iwata K, Phipps R, et al. Alterations in canine vertebral bone turnover, microdamage accumulation, and biomechanical properties following 1-year treatment with clinical treatment doses of risedronate or alendronate. Bone 2006;39:872–9.

36. Mashiba T, Turner CH, Hirano T, et al. Effects of suppressed bone turnover by bisphosphonates on microdamage accumulation and biomechanical properties in clinically relevant skeletal sites in beagles. Bone 2001;28:524–31.

37. Komatsubara S, Mori S, Mashiba T, et al. Suppressed bone turnover by long-term bisphosphonate treatment accumulates microdamage but maintains intrinsic material properties in cortical bone of dog rib. J Bone Miner Res 2004;19:999–1005.

38. Allen MR, Burr DB. Three years of alendronate treatment results in similar levels of vertebral microdamage as after one year of treatment. J Bone Miner Res 2007;22:1759–65.

39. Brennan O, Kennedy OD, Lee TC, et al. Effects of estrogen deficiency and bisphosphonate therapy on osteocyte viability and microdamage accumulation in an ovine model of osteoporosis. J Orthop Res 2011;29:419–24.

40. Boskey AL, Spevak L, Weinstein RS. Spectroscopic markers of bone quality in alendronate-treated postmenopausal women. Osteoporos Int 2009;20:793–800.

41. Donnelly E, Meredith DS, Nguyen JT, et al. Reduced cortical bone compositional heterogeneity with bisphosphonate treatment in postmenopausal women with intertrochanteric and subtrochanteric fractures. J Bone Miner Res 2012;27:672–8.

42. Roschger P, Rinnerthaler S, Yates J, et al. Alendronate increases degree and uniformity of mineralization in cancellous bone and decreases the porosity in cortical bone of osteoporotic women. Bone 2001;29:185–91.

43. Mashiba T, Hirano T, Turner CH, et al. Suppressed bone turnover by bisphosphonates increases microdamage accumulation and reduces some biomechanical properties in dog rib. J Bone Miner Res 2000;15: 613–20.

44. Allen MR, Iwata K, Sato M, et al. Raloxifene enhances vertebral mechanical properties independent of bone density. Bone 2006;39:1130–5.

45. Renders GA, Mulder L, van Ruijven LJ, et al. Mineral heterogeneity affects predictions of intratrabecular stress and strain. J Biomech 2011;44:402–7.

46. Viguet-Carrin S, Garnero P, Delmas PD. The role of collagen in bone strength. Osteoporos Int 2006;17: 319–36.

47. Oxlund H, Barckman M, Ortoft G, et al. Reduced concentrations of collagen cross-links are associated with reduced strength of bone. Bone 1995;17: 365S–71S.

48. Oxlund H, Mosekilde L, Ortoft G. Reduced concentration of collagen reducible cross links in human trabecular bone with respect to age and osteoporosis. Bone 1996;19:479–84.

49. Bailey AJ, Wotton SF, Sims TJ, et al. Post-translational modifications in the collagen of human osteoporotic femoral head. Biochem Biophys Res Commun 1992; 185:801–5.

50. Saito M, Mori S, Mashiba T, et al. Collagen maturity, glycation induced-pentosidine, and mineralization are increased following 3-year treatment with incadronate in dogs. Osteoporos Int 2008;19:1343–54.

51. Odetti P, Rossi S, Monacelli F, et al. Advanced glycation end products and bone loss during aging. Ann N Y Acad Sci 2005;1043:710–7.

52. Monnier VM, Sell DR, Abdul-Karim FW, et al. Collagen browning and cross-linking are increased in chronic experimental hyperglycemia. Relevance to diabetes and aging. Diabetes 1988;37:867–72.

53. Tang SY, Vashishth D. Non-enzymatic glycation alters microdamage formation in human cancellous bone. Bone 2010;46:148–54.

54. Vashishth D, Gibson GJ, Khoury JI, et al. Influence of nonenzymatic glycation on biomechanical properties of cortical bone. Bone 2001;28: 195–201.

55. Wang X, Shen X, Li X, et al. Age-related changes in the collagen network and toughness of bone. Bone 2002;31:1–7.

56. Tang SY, Zeenath U, Vashishth D. Effects of nonenzymatic glycation on cancellous bone fragility. Bone 2007;40:1144–51.

57. Tang SY, Allen MR, Phipps R, et al. Changes in nonenzymatic glycation and its association with altered mechanical properties following 1-year treatment with risedronate or alendronate. Osteoporos Int 2009; 20:887–94.

58. Lo JC, Huang SY, Lee GA, et al. Clinical correlates of atypical femoral fracture. Bone 2012;51:181–4.

59. Koh JS, Goh SK, Png MA, et al. Distribution of atypical fractures and cortical stress lesions in the femur: implications on pathophysiology. Singapore Med J 2011;52:77–80.

60. Tang WM, Chiu KY, Kwan MF, et al. Sagittal bowing of the distal femur in Chinese patients who require total knee arthroplasty. J Orthop Res 2005;23:41–5.

61. Food and Drug Administration. Background document for meeting of Advisory Committee for Reproductive Health Drugs and Drug Safety and Risk Management Advisory Committee. September 9, 2011. Available: (http://www.fda.gov/downloads/AdvisoryCommittees/CommitteesMeetingMaterials/Drugs/DrugSafetyandRiskManagementAdvisoryCommittee/UCM270958.pdf). Accessed on May 31, 2012.

62. Whitaker M, Guo J, Kehoe T, et al. Bisphosphonates for osteoporosis - where do we go from here? N Engl J Med 2012;366(22):2048–51.

63. Black DM, Bauer DC, Schwartz AV, et al. Continuing bisphosphonate treatment for osteoporosis - for whom and for how long? N Engl J Med 2012;366(22):2051–3.

64. Nancollas GH, Tang R, Phipps RJ, et al. Novel insights into actions of bisphosphonates on bone: differences in interactions with hydroxyapatite. Bone 2006;38: 617–27.

65. Vasikaran S, Eastell R, Bruyere O, et al. Markers of bone turnover for the prediction of fracture risk and monitoring of osteoporosis treatment: a need for international reference standards. Osteoporos Int 2011; 22:391–420.

66. Dell R, Greene D, Tran D. Stopping bisphosphonate treatment decreases the risk of having a second atypical femur fracture. Read at the annual meeting of the American Academy of Orthopaedic Surgeons. San Francisco, February 7–11, 2012.

67. Bischoff-Ferrari HA, Dawson-Hughes B, Willett WC, et al. Effect of vitamin D on falls: a meta-analysis. JAMA 2004;291:1999–2006.

68. Bischoff-Ferrari HA, Dietrich T, Orav EJ, et al. Higher 25-hydroxyvitamin D concentrations are associated with better lower-extremity function in both active and inactive persons aged >or =60 y. Am J Clin Nutr 2004;80:752–8.

69. Bischoff-Ferrari HA, Willett WC, Wong JB, et al. Fracture prevention with vitamin D supplementation: a meta-analysis of randomized controlled trials. JAMA 2005; 293:2257–64.

70. Tang BM, Eslick GD, Nowson C, et al. Use of calcium or calcium in combination with vitamin D supplementation to prevent fractures and bone loss in people aged 50 years and older: a meta-analysis. Lancet 2007;370:657–66.

71. Ross C, Taylor C, Yaktine A, et al. Dietary reference intakes for calcium and vitamin D. Washington, DC: National Academies Press; 2011. p. 1132.

72. Heaney RP, Holick MF. Why the IOM recommendations for vitamin D are deficient. J Bone Miner Res 2011;26:455–7.

73. Holick MF. Optimal vitamin D status for the prevention and treatment of osteoporosis. Drugs Aging 2007;24:1017–29.

74. Heaney RP, Davies KM, Chen TC, et al. Human serum 25-hydroxycholecalciferol response to extended oral dosing with cholecalciferol. Am J Clin Nutr 2003;77: 204–10.

75. Hollis BW. Circulating 25-hydroxyvitamin D levels indicative of vitamin D sufficiency: implications for establishing a new effective dietary intake recommendation for vitamin D. J Nutr 2005;135:317–22.

76. Hollis BW, Wagner CL. Normal serum vitamin D levels. N Engl J Med 2005;352:515–6 [author reply: 515–6].

77. Ettinger B, San Martin J, Crans G, et al. Differential effects of teriparatide on BMD after treatment with raloxifene or alendronate. J Bone Miner Res 2004; 19:745–51.

78. Gomberg SJ, Wustrack RL, Napoli N, et al. Teriparatide, vitamin D, and calcium healed bilateral subtrochanteric stress fractures in a postmenopausal woman with a 13-year history of continuous alendronate therapy. J Clin Endocrinol Metab 2011;96: 1627–32.

79. Andreassen TT, Ejersted C, Oxlund H. Intermittent parathyroid hormone (1-34) treatment increases callus formation and mechanical strength of healing rat fractures. J Bone Miner Res 1999;14:960–8.

80. Andreassen TT, Fledelius C, Ejersted C, et al. Increases in callus formation and mechanical strength of healing fractures in old rats treated with parathyroid hormone. Acta Orthop Scand 2001;72:304–7.

81. Skripitz R, Andreassen TT, Aspenberg P. Parathyroid hormone (1-34) increases the density of rat cancellous bone in a bone chamber. A dose-response study. J Bone Joint Surg Br 2000;82:138–41.

82. Zanchetta JR, Bogado CE, Ferretti JL, et al. Effects of teriparatide [recombinant human parathyroid hormone (1-34)] on cortical bone in postmenopausal women with osteoporosis. J Bone Miner Res 2003; 18:539–43.

83. Aspenberg P, Genant HK, Johansson T, et al. Teriparatide for acceleration of fracture repair in humans: a prospective, randomized, double-blind study of 102 postmenopausal women with distal radial fractures. J Bone Miner Res 2010;25:404–14.

84. Peichl P, Holzer LA, Maier R, et al. Parathyroid hormone 1-84 accelerates fracture-healing in pubic bones of elderly osteoporotic women. J Bone Joint Surg Am 2011;93:1583–7.

85. Cao Y, Mori S, Mashiba T, et al. Raloxifene, estrogen, and alendronate affect the processes of fracture repair differently in ovariectomized rats. J Bone Miner Res 2002;17:2237–46.

86. Martinez MD, Schmid GJ, McKenzie JA, et al. Healing of non-displaced fractures produced by fatigue loading of the mouse ulna. Bone 2010;46:1604–12.

87. Weil YA, Rivkin G, Safran O, et al. The outcome of surgically treated femur fractures associated with long-term bisphosphonate use. J Trauma 2011;71: 186–90.

88. Connolly JF, Guse R, Tiedeman J, et al. Autologous marrow injection as a substitute for operative grafting of tibial nonunions. Clin Orthop Relat Res 1991; 266:259–70.

89. Hernigou P, Mathieu G, Poignard A, et al. Percutaneous autologous bone-marrow grafting for nonunions. Surgical technique. J Bone Joint Surg Am 2006;88(Suppl 1 Pt 2):322–7.

90. Hernigou P, Poignard A, Beaujean F, et al. Percutaneous autologous bone-marrow grafting for nonunions. Influence of the number and concentration of progenitor cells. J Bone Joint Surg Am 2005;87: 1430–7.

91. Tiedeman JJ, Connolly JF, Strates BS, et al. Treatment of nonunion by percutaneous injection of bone marrow and demineralized bone matrix. An experimental study in dogs. Clin Orthop Relat Res 1991;268:294–302.

92. Tiedeman JJ, Garvin KL, Kile TA, et al. The role of a composite, demineralized bone matrix and bone marrow in the treatment of osseous defects. Orthopedics 1995;18:1153–8.

93. Saleh A, Hegde VV, Potty AG, et al. Management strategy for symptomatic bisphosphonate-associated incomplete atypical femoral fractures. HSS J 2012. http://dx.doi.org/10.1007/s11420-012-9275-y.

94. Koh JS, Goh SK, Png MA, et al. Femoral cortical stress lesions in long-term bisphosphonate therapy: a herald of impending fracture? J Orthop Trauma 2010;24:75–81.

Cognitive Dysfunction in Hip Fracture Patients

Harman Chaudhry, MD[a],*,
Philip J. Devereaux, MD, PhD, FRCPC[b,c],
Mohit Bhandari, MD, PhD, FRCSC[a]

KEYWORDS

- Cognitive dysfunction • Hip fracture • Delirium • Dementia

KEY POINTS

- Co-occurrence of cognitive dysfunction and hip fracture is common in elderly patients.
- Dementia is a chronic form of cognitive dysfunction that increases the risk of falling and sustaining a fracture; preventive efforts have therefore focused on reducing these risks.
- Delirium is an acute fluctuating state of confusion that is associated with worse functional outcomes, increased lengths of stay, morbidity, and mortality in patients with hip fractures.
- Preventive efforts surrounding delirium have focused on provision of specialized care, pharmacologic prophylaxis, pain management practices, and approaches to anesthesia.
- Conclusions are limited by the quality of available evidence. More high-level, adequately powered, and rigorously conducted prospective cohort studies and randomized controlled trials are needed.

Hip fractures represent a widespread morbidity among the geriatric population. In North America alone, more than 320,000 hip fractures are sustained annually, a number that is expected to increase as the population continues to age.[1,2] The impact of hip fractures on society in terms of associated morbidity, mortality (30-day mortality rate is 9% for men and 5% for women), and financial costs is staggering and will likewise continue to worsen.[3–5]

Disorders of cognition, primarily dementia and delirium, also have a higher-than-average incidence and prevalence among the geriatric population.[6] The co-occurrence of cognitive dysfunction and hip fracture is common and is an important entity for orthopedic surgeons and other clinicians involved in hip fracture care to recognize. Until recently, cognitive dysfunction in patients with hip fractures has been an issue that has received scant recognition compared with conditions considered to represent a more immediate threat to life, such as cardiopulmonary and thromboembolic diseases.[7]

This article reviews the currently available evidence surrounding cognitive dysfunction, specifically dementia and delirium, in patients with hip fractures.

METHODOLOGY

The MEDLINE database was searched for articles pertaining to dementia, delirium, or other cognitive disorders in patients with hip fractures. The following MeSH terminology was used: hip fracture AND [delirium OR dementia OR amnesia or delirium, dementia, amnestic, cognitive disorders]. The search was supplemented with searches of the PubMED database, EMBASE database, and reference lists of related articles. All article titles and abstracts were screened for

[a] Division of Orthopaedic Surgery, McMaster University, 293 Wellington Street North, Suite 110, Hamilton, Ontario L8L 8E7, Canada; [b] Department of Clinical Epidemiology and Biostatistics, McMaster University, 1280 Main Street West, Hamilton, Ontario L8S 4L8, Canada; [c] Department of Medicine, McMaster University, 1280 Main Street West, Hamilton, Ontario L8S 4L8, Canada
* Corresponding author.
E-mail address: chaudhh@mcmaster.ca

Orthop Clin N Am 44 (2013) 153–162
http://dx.doi.org/10.1016/j.ocl.2013.01.003
0030-5898/13/$ – see front matter © 2013 Elsevier Inc. All rights reserved.

relevance, and any uncertainty was resolved with screening of the full text of the article. The full text of all included articles was subsequently reviewed and the content organized thematically for this review.

DEMENTIA

Dementia is a syndrome characterized by persistent impairment in cognitive function as evidenced by deficits in short-term and long-term memory, attention, language, motor activity, and higher-level executive functions, such as problem solving. Many conditions may manifest as dementia, most of which are irreversible. As a chronic and often progressive condition, dementia may present on a spectrum of severity, ranging from mild cognitive impairment or "predementia" to advanced dementia.[8,9]

Magnitude of the Problem

Dementia is a prevalent condition in the hip fracture population. A recent meta-analysis of 34 studies published up to June 2009 found that the estimated prevalence of dementia in the literature pertaining to hip fracture is 19.2% (95% confidence interval, 11.4%–30.6%).[10]

Furthermore, individuals with dementia are more likely to fall, are more likely to fall repeatedly, and have a higher likelihood of sustaining a fracture secondary to fall, even when the number of falls are controlled for.[11–13] The reasons for this are likely multifactorial. Formiga and colleagues[13] showed that patients presenting with both hip fracture and dementia were more likely to have an intrinsic cause of fall, whereas those without dementia were more likely to have fallen secondary to extrinsic causes. This finding may be at least partially explained by cognitive impairment of patients with dementia, which results in gait disturbances. Studies have shown gait disturbances in patients with early executive function impairment.[14,15] In a recent 5-year prospective cohort study of 256 patients, investigators showed that even in the absence of dementia, early impairment in executive function was able to predict fall risk.[14] Furthermore, certain medications that patients with dementia are prescribed, such as anticholinergics, are also likely to precipitate syncope, falls, and hip fracture.[16]

In the context of hip fractures, dementia is relevant preoperatively as both a risk factor and a predictor of eventual outcome. Arguably, no conclusive evidence shows that dementia is acquired postoperatively, as recently summarized in a systematic review by Newman and colleagues.[17]

Diagnosis and Clinical Presentation

The diagnosis of dementia is clinical, with supplementary laboratory and imaging investigations required for workup of secondary potentially treatable causes. The diagnostic workup generally entails a clinical diagnosis of dementia, a thorough investigation for underlying causes of dementia, and the identification and management of contributory comorbidities.[18] The clinical diagnosis typically involves the use of brief cognitive tests, such as the Mini-Mental State Examination (MMSE), the Modified MMSE, or the Montreal Cognitive Assessment tool, to screen for cognitive impairment. These tools, among others, are fairly sensitive and specific in differentiating moderate dementia from normal cognitive function. However, they perform less than ideally in differentiating the milder forms of dementia and cognitive impairment.[18] Therefore, full neuropsychological testing is indicated in patients in whom mild dementia or cognitive impairment is suspected. Validated criteria, such as those presented in the fourth edition of the *Diagnostic and Statistical Manual of Mental Disorders* (DSM-IV), are then applied to consolidate the diagnosis.

A more comprehensive description and approach to the clinical presentation and diagnosis of dementia are beyond the scope of this review and readers are referred to other publications.[8,18]

Outcomes

Although it is well established that individuals with cognitive impairment and dementia are at increased risk of falls and fracture, whether these patients do worse when other comorbidities are controlled for in the short and long term after hip fracture is uncertain.

In a cohort of 348 patients studied retrospectively, Harboun and colleagues[19] found that patients with dementia are more likely to be institutionalized in the 3 years after a hip fracture than those who have not sustained a hip fracture.

Muir and Yohannes[20] performed a systematic review of the literature, which comprised 10 prospective cohort studies and 1 randomized controlled trial. Meta-analysis was not possible because of heterogeneity of outcomes. Studies included in this systematic review were evaluated to be of poor methodological quality. Sample sizes ranged from 48 to 320. The authors summarized findings pertaining to postfracture functional activity, length of stay, and discharge destination. No conclusive differences were evident in these studies between patients with and without prefracture dementia.

Patients with dementia at admission are more likely to develop delirium postoperatively.[21] The evidence and implications of this are discussed later in the Delirium section.

Overall, the postfracture implications of dementia have not been well elucidated in the scientific literature. Studies have generally been few in number and small in size, and lack standardization to allow for meta-analysis.

Prevention

As dementia is a chronic condition, prevention of dementia per se in the period immediately preceding hip fracture is not possible. In this context, preventive efforts pertaining to hip fracture involve preventing falls and subsequent fractures in this population.

Understanding factors leading to falls in patients with dementia is crucial to circumvention. Eriksson and colleagues[22] described the circumstances surrounding falls in patients with dementia on a psychogeriatric ward. They found no difference between the frequency of falls between day and night, although night falls were more likely to be unwitnessed. In terms of characteristics of the fall events, falls at night occurred more frequently off a platform, such as a chair or bed. Therefore, they were more likely to occur in the patient's room. Day falls were more likely to occur in a location outside the patient's room, such as a dining room or an activity area. Anxiety, darkness, and not wearing shoes were other risk factors for falls. In terms of characteristics of the patients, men were more likely to fall than women, and these falls were more likely to be associated with a delirious episode. When women fell, they were more likely to have an associated urinary tract infection than men. Given the nature of the study, causal mechanisms were impossible to identify.

The use of hip protectors is one intervention that has been studied as a possible means to prevent hip fracture secondary to fall. A recent prospective cohort study showed a lower rate of hip fractures among patients with dementia who wore hip protectors (relative risk, 5.63; number needed to treat, 28; P = .007).[23] However, the effectiveness of hip protectors in the community and institutional setting has been controversial, because several studies have not shown a benefit.[24] One study postulated that the lack of efficacy is predominantly secondary to a compliance issue. In this study by Garfinkel and colleagues,[23] compliance criteria were strict in an institutional setting, which probably contributed to the observed positive outcome. Therefore, hip protectors may be protective given appropriate patient and setting selection

to ensure adequate compliance, although making a firm suggestion in this regard is still controversial.[24] Randomized trials are needed to definitively inform the effect of this intervention.

Overall, evidence is insufficient to make any evidence-based recommendations regarding fall prevention in the dementia population. Optimal fall prevention strategies for patients with dementia are not well elaborated and further research is needed.

Treatment and Rehabilitation

After a hip fracture, one of the earliest and most important interventions that can be used is the relief of pain through adequate analgesia. Adequate pain control should be considered fundamental to the care of all patients with hip fractures, both as a moral and compassionate responsibility and because it can prevent secondary complications, such as the development of delirium. Unfortunately, pain control in patients with dementia is too frequently suboptimal despite evidence that these patients do experience pain.[25,26] A prospective study by Morrison and colleagues[27] comparing 59 cognitively intact patients with 38 patients experiencing dementia found that the latter group received one-third of the morphine sulfate equivalent as the former group. Most patients in either group did not receive a standing order for pain medication (arguably more important in patients with advanced dementia).[27] Part of the issue may be that health care personnel, such as nurses, are not adequately trained at assessing pain in patients with dementia.[28] Strategies could be considered, such as regular administration as opposed to as-needed administration.[27]

A nonblinded randomized controlled trial of 260 independent community-living patients in Finland was conducted to determine whether a specialized geriatric rehabilitation team consisting of physicians, nurses, and allied health professionals could impact length of stay, mortality, and place of residence at 3 months and 1 year.[29] An unequal distribution was seen based on MMSE scores postrandomization, and subgroup analyses were undertaken of the patients with and without low MMSE scores. Patients with hip fractures with mild to moderate dementia who received the intervention showed decreased length of stay and returned to independent community living at 3 months compared with controls. However, the significant difference did not persist at 1-year follow-up. The trial was not able to detect a significant difference in outcomes among patients with normal cognition and in those with severe dementia. Although no significant difference in mortality was detected, a trend was seen toward increasing mortality with increasing severity of dementia. This trial was certainly underpowered to detect a difference in its primary outcomes, because the a priori determined sample size of 250 was not achieved.

Patients with hip fractures who are not able to adequately regain function in the hospital are often discharged to specialized institutions for further rehabilitation. However, home-based rehabilitation is another option for community-dwelling patients with dementia after a hip fracture. In a prospective cohort study of patients with hip fractures managed operatively, Giusti and Barone[30] followed 55 patients discharged to a rehabilitation institution and 41 patients discharged directly home postoperatively. They found that function was at least equivalent to if not superior to institution-based rehabilitation as measured by the Barthel index for Activities of Daily Living (ADLs) and the Lawson index for Instrumental ADLs.[30]

DELIRIUM

Delirium is an acute state of confusion, which tends to have a short and fluctuating course but can last several weeks to months. It is characterized by the acuity of its onset (typically <24 hours), changes in level of consciousness, decreased ability to concentrate, cognitive decline, and perceptual disturbances.[31]

Magnitude of the Problem

Delirium is a condition especially prevalent in hospitalized patients. In certain hospital settings, its incidence is particularly marked. Next to patients admitted to the intensive care unit, postoperative patients and those with hip fractures are considered to be among those at the highest at risk for delirium.[32]

In regard to hip fracture, a meta-analysis of studies to 2005 showed a variable prevalence of delirium as reported in the orthopedic literature, ranging from 4.0% to 53.3%, with a pooled effect size of 21.7%. Consistently across studies, patients with hip fractures tended to have higher rates of postoperative delirium than those undergoing elective orthopedic surgery. Up to 35% of delirium cases were shown to have preoperative onset, a large proportion of which persisted postoperatively.[33]

Risk Factors and Causes

The pathophysiologic cause of delirium, although not completely understood, has been postulated to involve preexisting cerebral compromise secondary to aging or an underlying condition such as dementia. Subsequent insults by noxious external exposures result in further compromise and lead to the clinical manifestations of the delirious state. In accordance with this theory, clinical studies have generally attempted to elucidate patients at increased risk for delirium (preexisting compromise) or the external exposures that precipitate an episode of delirium.[31]

In an exploratory study, Juliebo and colleagues[34] studied many potential variables for possible predictive value of both preoperative and postoperative delirium. The investigators found that both precognitive impairment and sustaining an injury in an indoor environment were significantly more common in patients who developed delirium in hospital. Fever and lengthier waits for surgery were significantly correlated with preoperative delirium, whereas low body mass index (BMI) was significantly correlated with postoperative delirium. Because conclusions of causation or mechanism are impossible given the exploratory nature of this study, these results warrant further study.

In a prospective cohort study of 425 patients with hip fracture, Lee and colleagues[21] found that the risk factors for delirium were most relevant in the absence of dementia. Patients with dementia were at increased risk of developing delirium regardless of other risk factors (54% vs 26%; P<.001). Patients without dementia who were at increased risk of perioperative delirium were of advancing age (as a continuous variable), male sex, or low BMI, or had an operative time longer than 2 hours. Therefore, the authors noted that risk stratification must initially involve an assessment of preoperative cognitive status. This finding has been corroborated in other studies.[35,36]

Brauer and colleagues[37] had 571 cases reviewed by 2 physicians prospectively to determine precipitating causes of delirium. With well-defined prespecified diagnostic criteria, they were unable to determine a definitive cause of delirium in most cases. However, they did identify various factors that seemed to contribute to the development of postoperative delirium. Most commonly identified factors were sensory/environmental, infection, drugs, and fluid and electrolyte abnormalities.

Furlaneto and Garcez-Leme[38] more recently identified these same causative agents in the development of delirium in patients with hip fractures. However, in contrast to the study by Brauer and colleagues,[37] these investigators were able to identify a single underlying cause in most cases. However, a key limitation to this conclusion was that prespecified criteria for diagnosis were not defined. Therefore, their conclusions require cautious interpretation.

Diagnosis and Clinical Presentation

A diagnosis of delirium is made clinically at the bedside, with laboratory and imaging investigations supplementing the diagnosis through identifying an underlying correctable cause or ruling out other suspected diagnoses. The diagnosis is made when a patient meets accepted diagnostic criteria, such as those outlined by the DSM-IV (**Box 1**). Various assessment tools have been devised to assist with rapid assessment and diagnosis. Among these, the Confusion Assessment Method instrument is most widely used and has a high sensitivity and specificity for diagnosing delirium.[31] The MMSE has less than ideal sensitivity and specificity for diagnosing delirium.[31] Other instruments are available that rate the severity of dementia. These instruments are used frequently in research studies but rarely in the clinical setting.

Patients with delirium may present clinically with 1 of 3 subtypes: hyperactive, hypoactive, or mixed.[31] The patient with hyperactive delirium is often readily identifiable because of the heightened arousal manifested as aggression, agitation, and restlessness. Patients with hypoactive delirium typically are withdrawn, are lethargic, and have slowed psychomotor function. The diagnosis of delirium in these patients is frequently missed, because they are less likely to draw attention from nurses, physicians, and other health care practitioners. A mixed subtype presents with a variety of features of both hyperactive and hypoactive subtypes.

In a prospective cohort study of 103 patients presenting with hip fracture in a Swedish hospital, Duppils and Wikblad[39] observed certain prodromal behavioral changes that predicted subsequent development of delirium. Specifically, disorientation and urgent calls for attention were significantly associated with the development of delirium in hospital. One-third of these behavioral changes were seen between 25 to 48 hours before a patient was diagnosed with delirium. This study was likely underpowered to detect other pertinent prodromal behaviors. Trends were observed in other behaviors, such as increased psychomotor activity and perceptual disturbances, but were not able to achieve statistical significance. Furthermore, observations were not structured in this study, and therefore other important prodromal behaviors may have been missed.

Certain scales are available that identify a prodromal state that puts patients at risk of perioperative delirium. Using the Delirium Rating Scale-Revised-98 (DRS-R-98) in a prospective study of 101 patients at risk for postoperative delirium, investigators found that early elevations in scores as assessed by the scale were able to predict development of postoperative delirium. The authors suggested a possible role for structured postoperative observations in these patients.[40] Other scales have also been validated for detecting patients with hip fractures who are at high risk for developing delirium during hospital admission. Some examples include the Risk Model for Delirium Scale[41,42] and the NEECHAM confusion scale.[43] These tools have the potential to risk stratify patients for an appropriate increase in monitoring and intervention.

Outcomes

The literature has consistently shown that patients with delirium have poorer outcomes than those without delirium, showing higher rates of morbidity and mortality. This finding has been corroborated in patients with hip fractures, alongside increased lengths of hospital stay and functional decline. Resultant cognitive impairments after the resolution of delirium may never completely improve and also may have long-term implications.

Gruber-Baldini and colleagues[44] measured incident cognitive impairment in 673 community-dwelling patients with hip fractures and found that it resulted in sustained cognitive impairments (as measured by the MMSE) and declines in both ADLs and instrumental ADLs at 2 and 12 months after discharge from hospital.

Box 1
Diagnostic criteria for delirium[a]

1. Disturbance of consciousness, with reduced ability to focus, sustain, or shift attention.

2. Change in cognition or development of perceptual disturbance, which is not better accounted for by a preexisting or evolving dementia.

3. Disturbance develops over a short period (typically hours to days) and has a fluctuating course throughout the day.

4. Clinical evidence shows that the disturbance is attributable to the direct consequences of a general medical condition.

[a] All criteria must be met for diagnosis.
Adapted from Diagnostic and statistical manual of mental disorders, 4th edition, Text Revision (DSM-IV-TR). Washington, DC: American Psychiatric Association; 2000.

Krogseth and colleagues[45] also found long-term deterioration of cognitive function in patients with hip fracture. In a prospective cohort study after 106 patients with hip fracture without pre-fracture dementia, the investigators found that patients who had dementia at 6 months after hip fracture were significantly more likely to have experienced a delirious episode in hospital. Whether the delirium was simply a deterioration of preexisting cognitive dysfunction or was causally related to the subsequent dementia remains unclear.

A prospective cohort study of 682 elderly patients with no cognitive impairment at admission found lower rates of ADLs and ability to walk 10 feet, and higher rates of depressive symptoms and cognitive impairment up to 2 years postoperatively in patients who developed delirium preoperatively.[46] Edelstein and colleagues[47] also found higher rates of 1-year mortality, functional decline, and decline in independence in 47 community-dwelling patients who developed delirium after admission for hip fracture. Based on these studies, the literature suggests that patients with hip fractures who develop delirium tend to have poorer outcomes than those who do not develop delirium.

Some suggestion has been made that delirium can vary in severity and is not a dichotomous state. Marcantonio and colleagues[48] used the Memorial Delirium Assessment Scale to classify patients into mild or severe delirium and also to subclassify delirium into hyperactive or hypoactive subtypes. They found that patients with mild delirium fared better than those with severe delirium, as measured by nursing home placement and mortality at 6 months. They also found that any hyperactive component to delirium led to worse outcomes using the same measures. Finally, and interestingly, they discovered that patients who had subsyndromal delirium (ie, some symptoms of delirium but not an adequate number to fulfill criteria for diagnosis) also had outcomes as poor, and sometimes poorer, than those with mild delirium.

Delirium itself can persist for prolonged periods and its persistence may also negatively influence outcomes. Lee and colleagues[36] performed a prospective cohort study of 232 elderly patients with hip fracture managed operatively and found that delirium lasting longer than 4 weeks was associated with increased mortality at 2 years compared with patients with delirium lasting less than 4 weeks. Significant functional decline with prolonged delirium was also observed, as measured based on ability to ambulate independently outside one's home.

Prevention

Unlike dementia, delirium is an acute condition, and therefore acute prevention is feasible. Research on preventing delirium in patients with hip fractures has focused on interventions that decrease both the incidence and severity of delirium. The most effective interventions have involved provision of specialized care, although some research has evaluated pharmacologic prophylaxis, pain management practices, and approaches to anesthesia.

A prospective cohort study with a historical control group investigated whether the introduction of specialized geriatric nurses for patients with hip fractures would benefit those identified as being at high risk of delirium according to the NEECHAM confusion scale.[49] Sixty patients underwent the intervention, whereas 60 received usual care. This study found that involvement of geriatric nurses was not able to reduce the incidence of delirium, but was able to reduce the severity and length of delirium when it did occur. No effects on functional status or mortality were evident.

A randomized trial of 126 patients, allocating groups to either usual care or a proactive geriatrics consultation, found that early involvement of a geriatric physician who managed patients using a structured recommendation protocol could reduce the incidence and severity of delirium in patients hospitalized for hip fracture.[50]

In a nonrandomized experimental design, Deschodt and colleagues[51] assigned 287 patients to receive either usual care or care by a comprehensive inpatient geriatric consultation team consisting of a nurse, geriatrician, social worker, physiotherapist, and occupational therapist, all of whom specialized in geriatric care. The consultation commenced preoperatively and followed the patients until discharge. The investigators found that the incidence of postoperative delirium and cognitive decline at discharge was reduced in patients treated by the inpatient geriatric team. In patients who developed delirium, the severity did not differ between groups.

Bjorkelund and colleagues[52] implemented a comprehensive multifactorial intervention targeting key risk factors for delirium in the prehospital and perioperative settings. In this prospective cohort study of cognitively intact patients presenting with hip fracture, 131 patients experiencing the intervention were compared with a historical control cohort of 132 patients. The intervention group received a protocol-led intervention consisting of supplemental oxygen; intravenous fluids and extra nutrition; increased monitoring of vitals and other physiologic parameters; adequate pain relief; avoidance of transfer delays; daily screening for delirium; and avoidance of polypharmacy. The investigators detected a decrease in the incidence of postoperative delirium, from 34% to 22% ($P = .03$).

Studies have also examined pharmacologic prophylaxis for delirium. Kalsivaart and colleagues[53] performed a randomized controlled trial of 430 patients. The intervention consisted of 1.5 mg/d of haloperidol started preoperatively until postoperative day 3. The control group received a placebo with identical parameters. The study found that although the incidence of delirium did not decrease, the intervention significantly decreased its severity (as measured by the validated DRS-R-98), the length of delirium (5.4 vs 11.8 days), and also the length of hospital stay overall (17.1 vs 22.6 days). Currently, another group of investigators are evaluating melatonin as a possible prophylactic option, because it has been shown to decrease the incidence of delirium in medical and elective surgical patients.[54]

Adequate control of pain is important to the prevention of delirium. A prospective study of 541 patients showed that severe pain in cognitively intact patients with hip fractures was significantly associated with the development of delirium. In patients with cognitive impairment, pain could not be adequately assessed. However, low or absent use of opioid medication was significantly associated with the development of delirium after a hip fracture.[55] Meperidine was shown to increase rates of delirium among all patients, and it was recommended that it be avoided in the hip fracture population. Nie and colleagues[56] recently published their findings that poor pain control in Chinese patients with hip fracture has also been associated with increased risk of delirium.

Owing to the association between pain and postoperative delirium in patients with hip fractures, a randomized placebo-controlled trial attempted to elucidate whether a nerve block (fascia iliaca block) could help reduce the incidence of delirium in patients at intermediate or high risk of this complication.[57] The trial randomized 219 patients at intermediate or high risk for the development of delirium and found that these patients had a reduced incidence of delirium with the use of the fascia iliaca nerve block. Severity and duration of delirium were also decreased in the intervention group. Subsequent subgroup analysis found that this benefit was specific to intermediate-risk patients only; however, the number of participants considered at high risk was low (33 total), and therefore the study may have been underpowered to detect a true difference in this subpopulation.

Several studies have examined the role of anesthesia in the development of delirium in patients with hip fractures. A small cohort study of 34 patients with hip fractures from Brazil found that the use of midazolam was associated with an increased risk of delirium.[58] This finding is consistent with other research showing that benzodiazepines are associated with delirium.[59] In a prospective cohort of 236 patients with hip fractures, Sieber and colleagues[60] found no association between the type or dose of anesthetic or associated opioid use and delirium. A randomized controlled trial conducted by the same group randomized 114 patients undergoing hip fracture repair with spinal anesthesia to receive either light or deep sedation with propofol. The investigators found that depth of sedation was able to predict postoperative delirium. Specifically, lighter sedation was able to decrease the incidence of postoperative delirium from 40% to 19% ($P = .02$).[61] Depth of sedation in this study was monitored with electroencephalogram, which is not standard practice in most operating rooms. Dosage of propofol use was not found to be associated with the development of delirium.

Overall, available evidence suggests a proactive approach to the prevention and treatment of delirium. Patients should be risk stratified at admission and followed by trained nurses and specialized multidisciplinary geriatric teams. Adequate pain control is of importance, with early evidence suggesting regional anesthesia and optimal use of opioids as 2 potential components to the prevention of delirium. Corroboration of these findings with well-designed, adequately powered randomized controlled trials is required.

SUMMARY

Cognitive dysfunction in patients with hip fractures most commonly manifests as either dementia or delirium. Dementia is a chronic form of cognitive dysfunction that is common in the hip fracture population. It heavily predisposes to falls and subsequent fracture among elderly patients. Preventive efforts in this population of patients have focused on identifying risk factors and causes of falls. Although hip protectors have shown some promise in preventing hip fractures after a fall, appropriate patient selection, setting selection, and high rates of compliance are integral to success. Management of patients with hip fractures and dementia requires adequate pain control and specialized rehabilitation, whether in an institutional setting or at home.

Delirium is an acute confusional state that frequently develops in patients with hip fractures who are exposed to certain external precipitants. Diagnosis is clinical and may be preceded by a prodromal phase. Length of stay, functional recovery, morbidity, and mortality outcomes are worse in patients who develop delirium, and possibly exist on a continuum based on severity and length of delirium. Efforts at preventing incidence and reducing the severity of delirium have focused on early and active involvement of specialized geriatric personnel and protocols, adequate pain control, and optimal use of regional anesthesia.

This article attempts to provide a panoramic narrative overview of the available evidence pertaining to cognitive dysfunction in patients with hip fracture. Ultimately, the conclusions are limited by the quality of the available evidence. Most studies were observational, using either concurrent or historical control groups, and therefore could not control for all sources of potential bias. Future observational studies must be large enough to detect true differences in outcomes, and must strive to control for possible confounding variables. Arguably, without high-quality and consistent observational data, the true impact of cognitive dysfunction on patients with hip fractures cannot be comprehended. Therefore, a large prospective cohort study with close and meticulous follow-up is warranted to help practitioners truly understand all of the factors associated with outcome after hip fracture. Through delineating the relative and absolute impact of cognitive dysfunction on patients with hip fractures, its prognosis, prevention, and management can be better prioritized for targeted intervention.

The few clinical trials in the literature that have evaluated potential interventions are generally not randomized, not blinded, and underpowered. The randomized controlled trial is the gold standard in the hierarchy of evidence-based medicine when evaluating therapeutic questions. Therefore, the authors recommend that investigators aim to evaluate future interventions through the use of adequately powered and rigorously conducted randomized controlled trials. This strategy will enable the formation of a rigorous evidence base that can better inform future practice and policy, ultimately improving the care of patients with hip fractures and cognitive dysfunction.

REFERENCES

1. Bhandari M, Devereux PJ, Tornetta P 3rd, et al. Operative management of displaced femoral neck fractures in elderly patients: an international survey. J Bone Joint Surg Am 2005;87:2122–30.

2. Cooper C, Campion G, Melton LJ. Hip fractures in the elderly: a world-wide projection. Osteoporos Int 1992;2:285–9.

3. Brauer CA, Coca-Perraillon M, Cutler DM, et al. Incidence and mortality of hip fractures in the United States. JAMA 2009;302:1573–9.

4. Haentjens P, Autier P, Barette P, et al. Belgian hip fracture study group. The economic cost of hip fractures among elderly women. A one-year, prospective, observational cohort study with matched-pair analysis. J Bone Joint Surg Am 2001;83:493–500.

5. Johnell O, Kanis JA. An estimate of the worldwide prevalence, mortality and disability associated with hip fracture. Osteoporos Int 2004;15:897–902.

6. Ferri CP, Prince M, Brayne C, et al. Global prevalence of dementia: a Delphi consensus study. Lancet 2005;17:2112–7.

7. Robertson BD, Robertson TJ. Postoperative delirium after hip fracture. J Bone Joint Surg Am 2006;88:2060–8.

8. Forlenzo OV, Diniz BS, Gattaz WF. Diagnosis and biomarkers of predementia in Alzheimer's disease. BMC Med 2010;8:89.

9. Mitchell SL, Teno JM, Kiely DK, et al. The clinical course of advanced dementia. N Engl J Med 2009;361:1529–38.

10. Seitz DP, Adunuri N, Gill SS, et al. Prevalence of dementia and cognitive impairment among older adults with hip fractures. J Am Med Dir Assoc 2011;12:556–64.

11. Guo Z, Wills P, Viitanen M, et al. Cognitive impairment, drug use, and the risk of hip fracture in persons over 75 years old: a community-based prospective study. Am J Epidemiol 1998;148:887–92.

12. Van Doorn C, Gruber-Baldini AL, Zimmerman S, et al. Dementia as a risk factor for falls and fall injuries among nursing home residents. J Am Geriatr Soc 2003;51:1213–8.

13. Formiga F, Lopez-Soto A, Duaso E, et al. Characteristics of fall-related hip fractures in community-dwelling elderly patients according to cognitive status. Aging Clin Exp Res 2008;20:434–8.

14. Mirelman A, Herman T, Brozgol M, et al. Executive function and falls in older adults: new findings from a five-year prospective study link fall risk to cognition. PLoS One 2012;7:e40297.

15. Ble A, Volpato S, Zuliani G, et al. Executive function correlates with walking speed in older persons: the InCHIANTI study. J Am Geriatr Soc 2005;53:410–5.

16. Gill SS, Anderson GM, Fischer HD, et al. Syncope and its consequences in patients with dementia receiving cholinesterase inhibitors: a population-based cohort study. Arch Intern Med 2009;169:867–73.

17. Newman S, Stygall J, Hirani S, et al. Postoperative cognitive dysfunction after noncardiac surgery:

a systematic review. Anesthesiology 2007;106: 572–90.

18. Feldman HH, Jacova C, Robillard A, et al. Diagnosis and treatment of dementia: 2. diagnosis. CMAJ 2008;178:825–36.

19. Harboun M, Dorenlot P, Cohen N, et al. Impact of hip fracture, heart failure and weight loss on the risk of institutionalization of community-dwelling patients with dementia. Int J Geriatr Psychiatry 2008;23: 1245–52.

20. Muir SW, Yohannes AM. The impact of cognitive impairment on rehabilitation outcomes in elderly patients admitted with femoral neck fracture: a systematic review. J Geriatr Phys Ther 2009;32: 24–32.

21. Lee HB, Mears SC, Rosenberg PB, et al. Predisposing factors for postoperative delirium after hip fracture repair in individuals with and without dementia. J Am Geriatr Soc 2011;59:2306–13.

22. Eriksson S, Strandberg S, Gustafson Y, et al. Circumstances surrounding falls in patients with dementia in a psychogeriatric ward. Arch Gerontol Geriatr 2009;49:80–7.

23. Garfinkel D, Radomislsky Z, Jamal S, et al. High efficacy for hip protectors in the prevention of hip fractures among elderly people with dementia. J Am Med Dir Assoc 2008;9:313–8.

24. Rubenstein LZ. Hip protectors in long-term care: another confirmatory trial. J Am Med Dir Assoc 2008;9:289–90.

25. Cole LJ, Farrell MJ, Duff EP, et al. Pain sensitivity and fMRI pain-related brain activity in Alzheimer's disease. Brain 2006;129:2957–65.

26. Cole LJ, Gavrilescu M, Johnston LA, et al. The impact of Alzheimer's disease on functional connectivity between brain regions underlying pain perception. Eur J Pain 2011;15:568.e1–11.

27. Morrison RS, Siu AL. A comparison of pain and its treatment in advanced dementia and cognitively intact patients with hip fracture. J Pain Symptom Manage 2000;19:240–8.

28. Rantala M, Kankkunen P, Kvist T, et al. Post-operative pain management practices in patients with dementia – the current situation in Finland. Open Nurs J 2012;6:71–81.

29. Huusko TM, Karppi P, Avikainen V, et al. Randomised, clinically controlled trial of intensive geriatric rehabilitation in patients with hip fracture: subgroup analysis of patients with dementia. BMJ 2000;321: 1107–11.

30. Giusti A, Barone A. Rehabilitation after hip fracture in patients with dementia. J Am Geriatr Soc 2007;55: 1309–10.

31. Kaplan NM, Palmer BF. Etiology and management of delirium. Am J Med Sci 2003;325:20–30.

32. Spronk PE, Riekerk B, Hofhuis J, et al. Occurrence of delirium is severely underestimated in the ICU during daily care. Intensive Care Med 2009;35: 1276–80.

33. Bruce AJ, Ritchie CW, Blizard R, et al. The incidence of delirium associated with orthopedic surgery: a meta-analytic review. Int Psychogeriatr 2007;19: 197–214.

34. Juliebo V, Bjoro K, Krogseth M, et al. Risk factors for preoperative and postoperative delirium in elderly patients with hip fracture. J Am Geriatr Soc 2009; 57:1354–61.

35. Kagansky N, Rimon E, Naor S, et al. Low incidence of delirium in very old patients after surgery for hip fractures. Am J Geriatr Psychiatry 2004;12:306–14.

36. Lee KH, Ha YC, Lee YK, et al. Frequency, risk factors, and prognosis of prolonged delirium in elderly patients after hip fracture surgery. Clin Orthop Relat Res 2011;469:2612–20.

37. Brauer C, Morrison S, Silberzweig SB, et al. The cause of delirium in patients with hip fracture. Arch Intern Med 2000;160:1856–60.

38. Furlaneto ME, Garcez-Leme LE. Delirium in elderly individuals with hip fracture: causes, incidence, prevalence, and risk factors. Clinics (Sao Paulo) 2006;61: 35–40.

39. Duppils GS, Wikblad K. Delirium: behavioural changed before and during the prodromal phase. J Clin Nurs 2004;13:609–16.

40. De Jonghe JF, Kalisvaart KJ, Dijkstra M, et al. Early symptoms in the Prodromal Phase of delirium: a prospective cohort study in elderly patients undergoing hip surgery. Am J Geriatr Psychiatry 2007;15: 112–21.

41. Vochteloo AJ, Moerman S, van der Burg LS, et al. Delirium risk screening and haloperidol prophylaxis program in hip fracture patients is a helpful tool in identifying high-risk patients, but does not reduce the incidence of delirium. BMC Geriatr 2011;11:39.

42. Moerman S, Truinebreijer WE, de Boo M, et al. Validation of a risk model for delirium in hip fracture patients. Gen Hosp Psychiatry 2012;34:153–9.

43. Duppils GS, Johansson I. Predictive value and validation of the NEECHAM Confusion Scale using DSM-IV criteria for delirium as gold standard. Int J Older People Nurs 2011;6:133–42.

44. Gruber-Baldini AL, Zimmerman S, Morrison RS, et al. Cognitive impairment in hip fracture patients: timing of detection and longitudinal follow-up. J Am Geriatr Soc 2003;51:1227–36.

45. Krogseth M, Wyller TB, Engedal K. Delirium is an important predictor of incident dementia among hip fracture patients. Dement Geriatr Cogn Disord 2011;31:63–70.

46. Dolan MM, Hawkes WG, Zimmerman SI, et al. Delirium on hospital admission in aged hip fracture patients: prediction of mortality and 2-year functional outcomes. J Gerontol 2000;55:M527–34.

47. Edelstein DM, Aharonoff GB, Karp A, et al. Effect of postoperative delirium on outcome after hip fracture. Clin Orthop Relat Res 2004;422:195–200.

48. Marcantonio E, Ta T, Duthie E, et al. Delirium severity and psychomotor types: their relationship with outcomes after hip fracture surgery. J Am Geriatr Soc 2002;50:850–7.

49. Milisen K, Foreman MD, Abraham IL, et al. A nurse-led interdisciplinary intervention program for delirium in elderly hip-fracture patients. J Am Geriatr Soc 2001;49:523–32.

50. Marcantonio ER, Flacker JM, Wright RJ, et al. Reducing delirium after hip fracture: a randomized trial. J Am Geriatr Soc 2001;49:516–22.

51. Deschodt M, Braes T, Flamaing J, et al. Preventing delirium in older adults with recent hip Fracture through multidisciplinary geriatric consultation. J Am Geriatr Soc 2012;60:733–9.

52. Bjorkelund KB, Hommel A, Thorngren KG, et al. Reducing delirium in elderly patients with hip fracture: a multi-factorial intervention study. Acta Anaesthesiol Scand 2010;54:678–88.

53. Kalsivaart KJ, de Jonghe JF, Bogaards MJ, et al. Haloperidol prophylaxis for elderly hip-surgery patients at risk for delirium: a randomized placebo-controlled study. J Am Geriatr Soc 2005;53:1658–66.

54. De Jonghe A, van Munster BC, van Oosten HE, et al. The effects of melatonin versus placebo on deliriumin hip fracture patients: study protocol of a randomised, placebo-controlled, double blind trial. BMC Geriatr 2011;11:34.

55. Morrison RS, Magaziner J, Gilbert M, et al. Relationship between pain and opioid analgesics on the development of delirium following hip fracture. J Gerontol 2003;58:76–81.

56. Nie H, Zhao B, Zhang YQ, et al. Pain and cognitive dysfunction are the risk factors of delirium in elderly hip fracture Chinese patients. Arch Gerontol Geriatr 2012;54:e172–4.

57. Mouzopoulos G, Vasiliadis G, Lasanianos N, et al. Fascia iliaca block prophylaxis for hip fracture patients at risk for delirium: a randomized placebo-controlled study. J Orthop Traumatol 2009;10:127–33.

58. Santos FS, Wahlund LO, Varli F, et al. Incidence, clinical features and subtypes of delirium in elderly patients treated for hip fractures. Dement Geriatr Cogn Disord 2005;20:231–7.

59. Marcantonio ER, Juarez G, Goldman L, et al. The relationship of postoperative delirium with psychoactive medications. JAMA 1994;16:1518–22.

60. Sieber FE, Mears S, Lee H. Postoperative opioid consumption and its relationship to cognitive function in older adults with hip fracture. J Am Geriatr Soc 2011;59:2256–62.

61. Sieber FE, Zakriya KJ, Gottschalk A, et al. Sedation depth during spinal anesthesia and the development of postoperative delirium in elderly patients undergoing hip fracture repair. Mayo Clin Proc 2010;85:18–26.

Hip Fracture Protocols
What Have We Changed?

Gregory J. Della Rocca, MD, PhD*, Brett D. Crist, MD

KEYWORDS

- Hip fracture • Geriatric fracture center • Hip fracture protocol • Multidisciplinary care

KEY POINTS

- Geriatric hip fracture is a common condition that is increasing in prevalence as the population ages.
- Geriatric patients with hip fracture often have multiple medical comorbidities that complicate their treatment and functional outcomes.
- Expedited surgical management of hip fractures in elderly patients is associated with improved outcomes and reduced early complications.
- Medical optimization of elderly patients with hip fractures before surgical management improves postoperative outcomes and long-term functional outcomes.
- Multiple models exist for care of geriatric patients with hip fracture.
- Early results indicate that protocol-driven, multidisciplinary care of geriatric patients with hip fractures appears to offer improved patient outcomes.

INTRODUCTION

Hip fractures represent one of the most common causes of hospital admission for elderly patients, and result in profound morbidity and mortality.[1] As the population ages, the burden of osteoporosis and of hip fractures is expected to increase substantially.[2] Care of the elderly patient with hip fracture is resource intensive, involving substantial costs as well as health care provider and family time, both in the United States[3] and elsewhere.[4,5] The annual cost of hip-fracture care in the United States for all age groups in 2004 was estimated at $9 billion.[6] Estimates are that total annual costs for hip-fracture care in the United States may escalate to $35 billion (in 2012 dollars, $16 billion in 1984 dollars) by the year 2040.[3]

Care of hip fracture traditionally has focused on stabilization of the fracture at the earliest possible opportunity. Early stabilization allows for pain control and patient mobilization. Many studies have demonstrated that delays of greater than 24 to 48 hours from injury result in an increased 1-year mortality rate in elderly patients with hip fractures[7–13]; this consideration, however, must be tempered by the fact that optimization of medical comorbidities is often necessary before successful surgical treatment of the hip fracture in elderly patients. Because many elderly patients with hip fracture have multiple comorbidities and often also have polypharmacy (administration of 6–9 drugs simultaneously),[14] they require close medical management. Perhaps it is not simply the delay to surgery that results in the increased 1-year mortality rate.

Comanagement of geriatric patients with hip fracture was originally developed in England many decades ago.[15–17] In most centers, however, elderly patients with hip fractures have normally been admitted to the orthopedic surgery services, with medical, cardiology, or geriatric consultation only as deemed necessary by the orthopedic surgeons. Over the past 20 years, however,

Department of Orthopaedic Surgery, University of Missouri, 1 Hospital Drive, N116, DC053.10, Columbia, MO 65212, USA
* Corresponding author.
E-mail address: dellaroccag@health.missouri.edu

Orthop Clin N Am 44 (2013) 163–182
http://dx.doi.org/10.1016/j.ocl.2013.01.009
0030-5898/13/$ – see front matter © 2013 Elsevier Inc. All rights reserved.

increasing attention has been paid to comanagement models of elderly patients with hip fracture, with intimate involvement of geriatricians in the preoperative and postoperative care of these patients. At some institutions, standardized care pathways have been developed, with encouraging results. This article discusses historical methods of care of elderly patients with hip fracture, the development of comanagement strategies for geriatric patients with hip fracture, and the evolution of hip-fracture care models as they exist today.

TRADITIONAL MANAGEMENT OF ELDERLY PATIENTS WITH HIP FRACTURE

Hip fractures are a common cause of morbidity and mortality in elderly patients. Patients who sustain fractures of the hip (femoral neck fractures or intertrochanteric fractures) after a fall from a standing height are considered to be osteoporotic by the World Health Organization.[18] The bulk of these patients are elderly and predominantly female.[18] Attendant with advanced age are comorbidities and polypharmacy, either of which may be the proximate cause of the fall that precipitates the hip fracture.[19–21] Nevertheless, the hip fracture itself is the factor that directly leads to hospital admission. That being stated, the focus of traditional care methods has been to repair the hip fracture as expeditiously as possible, and gives little emphasis to medical management of these patients or to the diagnosis and treatment of osteoporosis.

Fracture stabilization has been demonstrated to improve outcomes for elderly patients with hip fracture. Although nonoperative management of such patients has been advocated in the past (especially for nonambulatory patients),[22] and early results of hip-fracture fixation in elderly patients were very poor,[23] routine use of this management method has fallen into disfavor. Early evidence that operative management of elderly patients with hip fracture was effective in reducing mortality rates was published by Sherk and colleagues[24] in 1979, demonstrating that early mortality decreased from more than 50% to 28% with "prompt" surgical stabilization (within 72 hours in 46 of 53 patients). Nevertheless, these mortality rates remained shockingly high.

Multiple studies have examined the effect of delaying surgical repair on outcomes in elderly patients with hip fracture. Conflicting reports were prevalent before 1995. One report indicated that patients undergoing early (ie, less than 24 hours post injury) hip-fracture fixation were more likely to expire within 1 year than those undergoing

fixation 2 to 5 days after injury.[25] The recommendation was that serious medical conditions should be stabilized for 24 hours or more after injury before scheduling surgery. However, another report showed that patients with 2 or fewer (but not 3 or more) preexisting medical comorbidities had increased 1-year mortality rates with operative delays of more than 24 hours after admission.[26] Another report indicated that operative delay of greater than 24 hours resulted in an increased 1-year mortality rate, without controlling for medical comorbidities.[27] Yet another report showed a decreased 3-month mortality rate in patients with hip fracture who had an operative delay greater than 48 hours from admission.[28] To confuse matters further, another study demonstrated that there was no relationship between delays to surgical repair of hip fractures and mortality at 2 years.[29]

In an effort to arrive at a recommendation for hip-fracture surgeons, Zuckerman and colleagues[7] conducted a prospective study to examine the effect of delay to surgical repair of hip fractures on in-hospital complications and on 1-year mortality rates in patients who were ambulatory and lived independently before fracture. A total of 367 patients were studied, and surgical hip-fracture repair was performed within 48 hours in 267 of the patients. Operative delay beyond 2 days doubled the risk of 1-year mortality. However, controlling for age, sex, and medical comorbidities revealed that the increase in 1-year mortality associated with surgical delay was not significantly different from the rate in patients treated early. When controlling for medical comorbidities and American Society of Anesthesiologists (ASA) class, no differences in in-hospital complications were noted between patients who underwent expeditious hip-fracture repair versus those who had a delay of greater than 48 hours. Nevertheless, the investigators recommended that surgical repair of hip fractures should occur within 2 days of hospital admission to minimize 1-year mortality rates.

A more stringent recommendation for early hip-fracture fixation was subsequently made by Hamlet and colleagues,[8] who conducted a retrospective review of 168 patients with 171 hip fractures. Data were gathered on ASA class as well as mortality rates for these patients. One-year mortality was only 20% if hip fracture repair was accomplished within 24 hours of admission, and 50% if accomplished after a delay of more than 24 hours from admission. The relative risk of death within 1 year was 4.5-fold higher in the surgical delay group, irrespective of the ASA classification. The investigators concluded that mortality rates are lower for patients with hip fracture if fracture repair is accomplished within 24 hours.

The publication of multiple studies implying that surgical delays for elderly patients with hip fracture resulted in higher mortality rates had the (perhaps) unintended effect of prompting caregivers to rush such patients to the operating room, sometimes forgoing complete medical optimization. Questions were asked about whether patients are at higher risk of mortality if their medical comorbidities are not optimized before surgical repair, and whether the higher mortality rate for hip-fracture patients who undergo delayed repair is exclusively due to the surgical delay or is instead due to the extreme comorbidities that may have caused the surgical delay. Surgical delays may be the result of unnecessary medical testing. A retrospective study of 235 consecutive elderly patients with hip fracture seemed to reveal that cardiology testing beyond electrocardiography (adenosine stress thallium testing, 2-dimensional echocardiography, dobutamine stress echocardiography, or diagnostic cardiac catheterization) did little else besides increasing costs and increasing delays between hospital admission and surgical care of the hip fracture.[30] What, then, is needed for preoperative evaluation of elderly patients with hip fracture? Is surgical delay truly the variable that affects mortality?

To answer this question, Grimes and colleagues[31] reported on a retrospective, multicenter trial of 8383 patients with hip fractures treated between 1983 and 1993. Long-term mortality rate (of up to 18 years) was used as the primary outcome measure. Early mortality (within 30 days), formation of pressure ulcers, serious infection, myocardial infarction, and venous thromboembolism were considered secondary outcome measures. Surgery was delayed more than 24 hours after admission in 4578 patients, to optimize the patients' medical conditions. There was no increase in long-term mortality in patients who underwent surgical repair within 48 hours of admission, compared with patients who waited more than 96 hours. No association between time to surgery and early mortality, serious infection, myocardial infarction, or venous thromboembolism was noted. An increased risk of pressure-ulcer formation was noted in patients who had a surgical delay of 96 hours or longer. The investigators concluded that waiting for up to 72 hours did not affect patient outcomes significantly. Risk of pressure ulcers was increased with long delays, but these may be prevented by minimizing conditions under which patients might develop them (eg, careful

monitoring, frequent turns, special mattresses, and nutritional supplementation). Delaying surgery for optimization of the medical condition of a patient with hip fracture was suggested to be beneficial in some cases.

Traditional methods of management of hip fractures in geriatric patients involved admission of patients to the orthopedic surgical service, rapid surgical stabilization, and involvement of other medical services only as deemed necessary by the attending orthopedic surgeon. Multiple studies revealed correlations between shorter times to the operating room and increased 1-year survival rates for these patients (**Table 1**). These data may have prompted a headlong rush to the operating room for surgical treatment of these patients without considering that delays in operative management may have been necessary for medical optimization of the patients for surgery. Those patients delayed for longer periods may have an increased 1-year mortality rate owing to their overall medical condition, as opposed to simply the amount of time from fracture to surgical treatment. In recognition of these considerations, centers began considering the development of care pathways for geriatric patients with hip fracture, with the aim of improving long-term outcomes.

DEVELOPMENT OF CARE PATHWAYS AND COMANAGED CARE FOR ELDERLY PATIENTS WITH HIP FRACTURE

Geriatric patients with fracture provide layers of complexity in management that are often absent in the young patient. The geriatric patient not only desires a return to function but also generally desires a return to independence (or prefracture way of life). Involvement of multiple physician teams, each with different expertise, has come to be expected for the geriatric patient with fracture. Despite this, comanaged care models for geriatric patients with hip fracture are relatively new developments in the United States. Care pathways, however, have been used and examined in other countries, and have led to their development in the United States.

Geriatric orthopedics requires a good working relationship between medical and surgical specialists to achieve the most favorable outcomes. The idea of "total care," or application of geriatric medical and surgical skills from the time of admission to the hospital through patient discharge, was proposed as important in giving the geriatric patient with hip fracture the highest likelihood of returning to independence (prefracture state of living).[32] Emphasis is placed on total care of the elderly for the purposes of returning them to an

Table 1
Studies referencing "traditional" methods for the care of geriatric patients with hip fracture

Authors,[Ref.] Year	Country	Inclusion Criteria	Exclusion Criteria	Study Design	Conclusion Summary	Level of Evidence
Sherk et al,[24] 1979	USA	"Senile" elderly hip-fracture patients	None specified	Retrospective	Favors early stabilization, "early" and "prompt" not defined	IV
Kenzora et al,[25] 1984	USA	Hip-fracture patients	None specified	Retrospective	Favors surgical delay until medical condition is stabilized, 2–5 d	IV
Sexson and Lehner,[26] 1987	USA	Hip-fracture patients	None	Retrospective	Favors stabilization within 24 h of hospitalization if healthy, but delay for optimization of unhealthy patients is acceptable	IV
White et al,[27] 1987	Canada	Hip-fracture patients	Pathologic or "severe trauma" or loss to follow-up	Retrospective	Favors early stabilization, but considers that increased mortality in delayed patients was related to high surgical risk	IV
Davis et al,[28] 1988	Great Britain	Intertrochanteric fracture patients	<50 y old, unfit for anesthesia	Retrospective	Timing unimportant for outcome	IV

Study	Country	Population	Exclusions	Study Type	Conclusion	Level of Evidence
Davidson and Bodey,[29] 1986	Great Britain	Hip-fracture patients	None	Retrospective	No association between surgical delay and mortality	IV
Zuckerman et al,[7] 1995	USA	Hip fracture, ≥65 y old, live at home	Dementia, nonambulatory	Prospective	Favors stabilization within 2 d of hospitalization	I (prognostic)
Hamlet et al,[8] 1997	USA	Hip fracture	Fractures treated at different institution, nonoperatively managed fractures, polytraumatized patients, pathologic fractures	Retrospective	Favors stabilization within 24 h of hospitalization	IV
Ricci et al,[30] 2007	USA	Hip fracture, ≥60 y old	None	Retrospective	No conclusions regarding mortality; cardiac testing beyond electrocardiogram results in unacceptable surgical delay	IV
Grimes et al,[31] 2002	USA	Hip fracture, ≥60 y old, data available from previous transfusion study	Cancer, trauma, declined blood transfusion	Retrospective	Time unimportant for outcome	IV

independent, active life. One of the tenets described in the care of geriatric fracture is expeditious fracture stabilization, which allows for a more rapid return to independence. However, appropriate medical management of preexisting comorbidities, both preoperatively and postoperatively, is essential.

Implementation of care pathways for elderly patients with hip fracture has been analyzed extensively since the end of the twentieth century. A white paper from Great Britain's National Health Service in 1997 stressed the need for health care providers to work collaboratively on integrated care for geriatric patients with hip fracture.[33] Care pathways have been used successfully in multiple disciplines outside of hip-fracture care to improve care delivery for elderly patients. Examples of successful implementation of care pathways, both in the United States and elsewhere, include those for total hip arthroplasty,[34] acute coronary syndromes,[35] acute pediatric illnesses,[36] and vascular surgery.[37]

An early report regarding the use of care pathways for the treatment of elderly patients with hip fracture (in Canada) was published by Ogilvie-Harris and colleagues[38] in 1993. The prospective cohort study compared 51 patients treated in a standard fashion with 55 patients treated according to a care map. The care map included a daily summary of scheduled events along with time frames for their completion. The maps were developed collaboratively by physicians, nurses, therapists, social workers, and others (as necessary) involved with the patient's care, and included standardized order sets. The investigators reported a statistically significant difference in outcome, with more patients returning to prefracture ambulatory and living status. There were fewer postoperative complications, and a higher number of patients returned home within 2 weeks of hospital admission. There was a slight trend toward reduced length of stay in the care-map cohort (13.6 vs 15.3 days) if patients who required greater than 28 days of hospitalization were excluded from both groups.

In Australia, a clinical pathway for the management of elderly patients with hip fracture was successful in decreasing lengths of stay in hospital and rates of wound infection, without changes in unplanned patient readmission, walking ability before discharge, or destination after discharge. In this study, Tallis and Balla[39] reviewed a clinical management program that was implemented in 1993, and their study compared two cohorts of patients: one of 90 patients who were treated in the 6 months before program implementation, and another of 88 patients who were treated in the 6 months following program implementation. Patients were excluded from analysis if they were younger than 50 years, had metastatic disease, or had multiple fractures. The average length of stay for hip fracture patients treated with the clinical management program decreased to 11.0 days, from 19.3 days before program implementation (P<.0001).

Another study on the use of clinical pathways in the care of elderly patients with hip fractures[40] revealed similar findings to those of Tallis and Balla. In this prospective trial, 111 consecutive elderly patients with hip fracture were "pseudorandomized" to receive established standard-of-care treatment (56 patients) or clinical pathway–guided treatment (55 patients). Clinical-pathway patients had a shorter hospital length of stay (6.6 vs 8.0 days, P = .03), and there was no difference noted in complications and readmission rates between the two cohorts.

Health-related quality of life and patient satisfaction with care of hip fracture does not appear to suffer from use of a clinical pathway, despite the decreased time of hospitalization. A 12-month prospective cohort study of 57 elderly patients with hip fracture revealed decreased complications and a decreased average length of hospital stay (3.3 days) when a care pathway was implemented, with no decrease in health-related quality of life or patient-satisfaction measures.[41]

A large observational cohort study was published in 2000 by March and colleagues.[42] This multicenter study compared 455 elderly patients with hip fracture managed before implementation of a hip-fracture clinical pathway with 481 patients managed after implementation. The results showed a small reduction in average length of stay in hospital and an increased use of evidence-based best practices after implementation of the clinical pathway, without changes in 4-month mortality rates or residential status of the patients after discharge.

The New Zealand Guidelines group recently published an extensive set of recommendations regarding multidisciplinary care of the elderly patient with hip fracture.[43] These guidelines recommend that patients be admitted to a formal hip-fracture program that is either orthogeriatric or based in the orthopedic ward. The program should include orthogeriatric assessment, rapid surgical optimization, and identification of multidisciplinary rehabilitation goals for the hip-fracture patients such that the likelihood of returning to prefracture status is maximized. Also, multidisciplinary review of the patients should occur throughout the hospitalization. Liaisons should be in place to assist with prevention of falls, management of osteoporosis, social services, and mental health services.

As low-energy hip fractures in the elderly population are pathognomonic for a diagnosis of osteoporosis, incorporation of medical management of deficient bone density seems to be a reasonable component of a hip-fracture treatment pathway. In 2002, a report of 385 consecutive patients with low-energy fractures ("osteoporotic fractures") revealed that almost two-thirds of patients were prescribed osteoporosis management regimens, and that two-thirds of those patients were still compliant with treatment at 6 months.[44] Of note, treatment was based on results of dual x-ray absorptiometry testing, which is not currently reimbursable for inpatients in the United States. Nevertheless, incorporating osteoporosis management recommendations into a care pathway for hip fractures may prove to be beneficial for long-term outcomes.

Together, the aforementioned studies represent early evidence in favor of establishing care pathways for the treatment of elderly patients with hip fracture (**Table 2**). The studies demonstrated reduced lengths of stay, and some revealed reduced complications, with implementation of a written hip-fracture management protocol. Further interest in the development of clinical pathways for care of patients with hip fracture has stimulated an investigation of 4 distinct models of care for this frail patient population.

MODELS OF CARE FOR THE GERIATRIC PATIENT WITH HIP FRACTURE

Four distinct models for the care of geriatric patients with hip fracture (**Table 3**) have been described by Pioli and colleagues,[45] and reviewed more recently by Kammerlander and colleagues.[46] The first model, considered the simplest, is standard orthopedic management with consultation by geriatric medicine only as desired by the orthopedic team, and often only postoperatively (perhaps a traditional standard-of-care method that predated comanagement models in the United States). The second is orthopedic admission with daily geriatric consultation from admission through discharge. The third is geriatric admission with orthopedic consultation from admission through discharge. The fourth model involves fully integrated care of these patients whereby the orthopedic surgeon and geriatrician comanage the patient entirely from admission through discharge.

Orthopedic Management with Occasional Geriatric Consultation

A simple model for the care of geriatric patients with hip fracture is orthopedic admission, with geriatric consultation only as necessary. Geriatric consultation is obtained variably, based on preferences of the admitting orthopedic surgeon, and occasionally is only obtained for assistance in postoperative management. In a prospective, randomized trial, Kennie and colleagues[47] compared two groups, each with 54 elderly patients with hip fracture, with regard to postoperative rehabilitation. All patients in both groups were admitted to the orthopedic service, underwent fracture repair, and then were managed postoperatively on the orthopedic ward (control group) or were transferred to an orthopedic rehabilitation ward at a neighboring facility (treatment group). Patients in the treatment group received daily care by a general practitioner, with intermittent but regular input from a geriatrician. Compared with patients in the control group, patients in the treatment group were noted to be significantly more likely to return to activity of daily living independence and had a significantly shorter length of stay in hospital; they were also more likely to return to their own homes and less likely to be discharged to institutional care settings.

Another study of postoperative interdisciplinary care consultation demonstrated that postoperative interventions did not result in improved short-term outcomes.[48] Patients were randomized to receive interdisciplinary care (n = 141) or standard care (n = 138) after surgical repair of hip fractures. Interdisciplinary care included daily care by a geriatrician, physical and occupational therapists, nurse specialists, and social workers, and included twice-weekly rounds. There was no difference in the number of patients alive without decline in ambulatory status for either group. However, postoperative interdisciplinary care resulted in a longer hospital stay (29.2 days for the interdisciplinary group, 20.9 days for the standard-care group; $P<.001$), despite there being no differences between groups for length of institutional care after discharge (including inpatient rehabilitation).

The 2 aforementioned studies describe a sequence of admission to an orthopedic service, orthopedic surgical care, and postoperative management that involves varying degrees of input from geriatricians and rehabilitation teams. The intervention (postoperatively) resulted in shorter length of stay in hospital in one study and an increased hospital stay in the other. These

Table 2
Studies focusing on development of care pathways for elderly patients with hip fracture

Authors,[Ref.] Year	Country	Inclusion Criteria	Exclusion Criteria	Study Design	LOS	Mortality	Complications	Conclusion Summary	Level of Evidence
Ogilvie-Harris et al,[38] 1993	Canada	Elderly hip-fracture patients	None specified	Prospective	Significantly more patients in protocol group were discharged in <14 d (P = .047)	16% in control group, 9% in protocol group (P = .01[a])[b]	33% in control group, 18% in protocol group (P = .01[a])	Better outcome and fewer postoperative complications in group of patients treated with management protocol	II (therapeutic)
Tallis and Balla,[39] 1995	Australia	Hip-fracture patients	<50 y of age, multiple fractures, pathologic fracture	Retrospective	19.3 d preprotocol, 11.0 d postprotocol (P<.0001)	2% in control group, 3% in program group	No difference for systemic complications, wound infection higher in control group (6.7% vs 0%, P = .02)	Outcomes quality maintained while LOS dropped dramatically after implementation of a care protocol for hip-fracture patients	III (therapeutic)

Choong et al,[40] 2000	Australia	Hip-fracture patients managed surgically	No surgery or "non-standard" surgery	Prospective	8.0 d control, 6.6 d pathway (P = .03)	None reported	36% control, 24% pathway (P = .40)	Multidisciplinary care pathways for hip-fracture patients reduce LOS without increasing complications	II (therapeutic)
Santamaria et al,[41] 2003	Australia	Hip-fracture patients managed surgically	Pathologic fracture, dementia, unwilling to participate	Prospective	14.4 d control, 11.1 d pathway (P = .15)	One in each group (P = .48)	54% control, 48% pathway (P = .90)	Shorter LOS and reduced complications noted for hip-fracture patients after implementation of care pathway	Uncertain
March et al,[42] 2000	Australia	All hip-fracture admissions	None	Retrospective	11–11.5 d control, 9.0 d pathway (P<.01)	16.8% in control group at 3 mo, 17.6% in pathway group (P = .826)	"...pathway use was not associated with a lower rate of postoperative complications..."	Clinical pathway results in reduced LOS but has no effect on mortality or residential status	III (therapeutic)

Abbreviation: LOS, length of stay.

[a] P value indicated for entire cohort including morbidity and mortality groups.

[b] In-hospital mortality.

Table 3
Models for geriatric hip-fracture care

Model Type	Admitting Service	Consultation Type[a]	Automatic Consultation?
1	Orthopedic	Medical/geriatric	No
2	Orthopedic	Medical/geriatric	Yes
3	Medical/geriatric	Orthopedic	Yes
4	Geriatric and orthopedic	Not applicable	Not applicable

[a] Either medical/geriatric or orthopedic. Other consultations obtained on a case-by-case basis.

conflicting results are difficult to reconcile. Perhaps the patients in the second study were sicker than those in the first. Nevertheless, these reports represent some early forays into the idea of comanagement protocols for geriatric patients with hip fractures.

Orthopedic Management with Daily Geriatric Consultation

In the second model of care, orthopedic admission of patients with hip fracture is accompanied by daily geriatric consultative care. Multiple studies have examined this method of care.[6,49–53] The conflicting results of these studies, however, lead to an inability to make conclusions regarding the efficacy of this model.

In one small trial of 71 patients, a shorter length of stay in hospital was noted with an early intervention program involving daily therapy, daily monitoring of patient needs via a multidisciplinary team approach, early surgery, and minimization of narcotic use.[49] Patients were randomly assigned to standard care (control group, 33 patients) or to the intervention group (38 patients). Mean length of stay for the intervention group was 21 days, compared with 32.5 days for the control group (P<.01). No differences were noted between groups for in-hospital mortality.

A cohort study with historical controls was performed at a New York hospital after implementation of a "Geriatric Hip Fracture Program."[50] The program involved care of patients with hip fracture via a multidisciplinary team approach. The team included an orthopedic surgeon, an internist or geriatrician, an anesthesiologist, nurses with geriatric training, physical and occupational therapists, an ophthalmologist, a psychiatrist, a case manager, and social workers. A total of 431 Geriatric Hip Fracture Program patients were included in the study, and were compared with a matched cohort of 60 geriatric patients with hip fracture treated before the initiation of the program. The investigators saw a decrease in transfers to the intensive care unit, improved ambulation, fewer

postoperative complications, and fewer discharges to nursing facilities. However, lengths of stay were not significantly different between the groups (23.2 days for the program group, 27.7 days for the control group).

The same group subsequently published on the implementation of a clinical pathway for elderly patients with hip fracture.[6] Standardized steps in care were delivered at each stage of the patient's admission, including preoperative supportive care and thromboembolic prophylaxis, optimization for surgery, preparation for surgery, postoperative care, and discharge. A comparison was made between 747 elderly patients with hip fracture treated before implementation of the clinical pathway (control group) and 318 patients treated after its implementation (clinical pathway group). The results showed significant decreases in length of stay in hospital (21.6 vs 13.7 days, P<.001), in-hospital mortality (5.3% vs 1.5%, P<.001), and 1-year mortality (14.1% vs 8.8%, P<.01) for the clinical pathway group in comparison with the control group.

Development of an integrated care pathway for the treatment of elderly patients with hip fracture was reported by Roberts and colleagues.[51] The specifics of this pathway are not delineated, but they state that the team was multidisciplinary. The investigators compared a prepathway cohort (400 patients) with a pathway cohort (381 patients), and noted an increase in length of stay of 6.5 days after implementation of the integrated care pathway (P<.0005). However, they also reported significantly increased ability to ambulate at time of discharge, and a trend toward reduced admission to a long-term care facility.

Fisher and colleagues[52] described a method of orthopedic and geriatric medicine "cocare" that involved daily oversight of medical care by a geriatric medical registrar and a weekly geriatric consultant review. Five hundred four geriatric patients with hip fracture managed before the geriatric medicine cocare program (historical controls) were compared with 447 patients managed after the introduction of the program (prospective cohort). There was a significant decrease in post-operative medical complications and mortality rate, as well as 6-month rehospitalization rate, after implementation of the cocare program. Length of stay in both cohorts was not significantly different. Substantial increases in the use of anti-osteoporotic treatment and thromboprophylaxis after implementation of cocare were also noted.

Cogan and colleagues[54] presented a retrospective cohort study of elderly patients with hip fracture admitted to a single hospital in Dublin, Ireland. Two cohorts of patients were compared: 103 patients admitted in 2001, before the appointment of a part-time, consulting senior registrar in geriatric medicine, and 98 patients admitted in 2006, after the appointment of the geriatric consultant. In 2006, the geriatric consultant performed a comprehensive geriatric assessment during the first 2 days of patient admission, and there were weekly multidisciplinary meetings with the geriatric consultant, surgeons, therapists, nurses, and social workers. The results showed a decrease in inpatient mortality from 20% to 8%, a decrease in nursing-facility discharges from 25% to 21%, and an increase in discharges directly to home from 8% to 18%, from the 2001 cohort to the 2006 cohort. Moreover, deep venous thrombosis prophylaxis, perioperative antibiotics, and osteoporosis medications were used more routinely in the 2006 cohort.

Despite successful implementation of daily geriatric consultation for elderly patients with hip fracture, as presented in the aforementioned publications, results are not always substantially improved over orthopedic care with geriatric consultation only as requested by the orthopedic surgeon. A prospective cohort study of 745 elderly patients with hip fracture conducted over 5 years revealed no significant improvements on mortality, length of stay, or discharge destination after implementation of "orthogeriatric care," whereby a geriatrician comanaged the patients jointly with orthopedic surgeons.[53] Despite a lack of evidence in this study that orthogeriatric care was of benefit to patients with hip fracture, the investigators stated that there was a perceived improvement in confidence in the anesthesia and orthopedic teams in the management of these patients after involvement of the geriatrician.

The second model of care for geriatric hip fractures, orthopedic admission with daily geriatric consultation, resulted either in improvement of care (as assessed by decreased hospital lengths of stay, decreased 1-year mortality rates, and decreased early complication rates)[6,49,50,52,54] or in overall improvement in confidence in managing these patients despite a lack of substantive measures of care improvement.[51,53] However, some physicians are of the opinion that the hip fracture, while the proximate cause of admission of hip-fracture patients, does not represent the main patient problem; rather, the hip fracture may be a result of the comorbid conditions. Therefore, some clinicians have advocated the admission of geriatric patients with hip fracture to geriatric medical services with orthopedic consultation, as described now.

Geriatric Management with Daily Orthopedic Consultation

In this model of care, elderly patients with hip fracture are admitted to the geriatric ward/service, and orthopedic care is provided on a consultation basis. This model has been adopted at several centers, including the University of Missouri. Although published studies that have investigated this model of care are limited, results pooled from all studies show inconsistent improvements after implementation of the model (when compared with premodel standards of care).[55–59]

In 1978 in Nottingham, England, an orthogeriatric unit was established in which elderly patients with hip fracture were managed in a unit run jointly by an orthopedic trauma service and the Department of Health Care of the Elderly.[58] After the unit was opened, there was a substantial increase in hip-fracture admissions. A substantial decrease in length of stay in hospital was noted from the year before the unit opened (66 days) to the year after it opened (48 days).

In 1983, an orthopedic geriatric unit was established at Gartnavel General Hospital (Glasgow, Scotland), in which geriatric medical, nursing, and allied health professional staff was provided. This randomized controlled trial of female patients with hip fracture aged 65 years or older demonstrated that mortality, length of stay, and discharge destination were all similar between the two groups of patients: one treated on the orthopedic ward (125 patients) and the other treated in the orthopedic geriatric unit (97 patients).[55] However, there was a notable increase in the diagnosis and treatment of medical comorbidities in patients in the orthopedic geriatric unit (71% new diagnoses) compared with the control group (55% new diagnoses) ($P<.025$).

A prospective study of 320 consecutive elderly patients admitted for hip fracture at a single hospital in Israel revealed improvements in patient care and outcomes for those treated in an orthogeriatric setting in comparison with orthopedic care followed by geriatric rehabilitation.[57] The cohort of patients was divided into two groups: 204 patients were admitted to the orthopedic ward, underwent surgery, and were subsequently transferred to the orthogeriatric ward for rehabilitation, and 116 patients were admitted to the orthogeriatric ward, where they received care from admission through surgery and rehabilitation. Ward assignment was exclusively based on bed availability on the orthogeriatric ward. Despite patients in the orthopedic-ward group being younger and less cognitively impaired than patients in the orthogeriatric-ward group, patients were more likely to rehabilitate successfully if managed exclusively on the orthogeriatric ward ($P = .03$), as assessed using objective outcomes instruments.

A follow-up study from Israel described results using the Sheba model of orthogeriatric care for elderly patients with hip fracture.[59] This model is based on the theory that hip fracture is the result of geriatric comorbidities rather than the primary disease. All surgical, medical, and rehabilitative requirements are managed in a single geriatric-oriented unit. The study reviewed 592 consecutive patients managed with this model. The results demonstrated low rates of mortality, short hospital stays, and good functional outcomes. A limitation of this study is the lack of a control group, although the results compare favorably with those of other published studies.

A randomized controlled trial of 199 patients with femoral neck fracture older than 69 years revealed that multidisciplinary postoperative care increased mobility and ability to accomplish activities of daily living in both short-term (4 months) and long-term (12 months) settings.[56] Of importance in this study was that only postoperative care was multidisciplinary. Preoperative care was conventional, on the orthopedic ward. Nevertheless, integrated postoperative care appeared to offer encouraging results for elderly patients with hip fracture in the near term (12 months) following hip-fracture repair.

Admission to a medical service with orthopedic consultation demonstrated encouraging results in the aforementioned studies. The model seems to be a reasonable extension of the thought that a geriatric patient with a hip fracture has comorbidities that cause the fracture, and the fracture is merely the factor that leads to hospital admission. Despite the encouraging results, this method of hip-fracture care may be less attractive to the geriatric services than is admission to an orthopedic service with geriatric consultation. At some centers, volumes of patients with hip fracture may be large enough that a geriatric admitting service could be overwhelmed with patients. Also, some disparities remain between billings and collections for evaluation and management services provided as part of an admission and ongoing hospital care as opposed to consultation (with the latter billing higher). Finally, the geriatricians may believe that the patient's true problem remains the orthopedic problem: the fracture itself. Perhaps a care pathway that exhibits a true comanagement mechanism might be beneficial. In this manner, geriatricians and orthopedic surgeons would share all aspects of responsibility for a patient's care, in a coordinated fashion; this represents the fourth model of care.

Fully Integrated Orthopedic and Geriatric Care

The 3 models of care already discussed for elderly patients with hip fracture all involve a primary service, either orthopedic surgery or geriatrics, with consultation from the other service. A true comanagement model, however, in which both services (plus other disciplines) are fully integrated in the care patients, is a relatively new development. Principles of this type of model have been summarized very well by Friedman and colleagues,[60] and are based on a model developed at the University Hospitals of Cleveland called the Acute Care for Elders unit (ACE unit).[61] At Highland Hospital (Rochester, NY) a geriatric fracture center has been established, following ACE unit guidelines. The principles of management for the geriatric fracture center have been enumerated as follows: the bulk of patients with hip fracture should undergo surgical stabilization, iatrogenic illnesses (eg, pressure ulcers, pneumonia, thromboembolic disease) are minimized by early surgery and true comanagement (geriatric and orthopedic service "co-ownership"), standardized protocols minimize missed steps in management that could lead to adverse outcomes, and discharge planning should begin at the time of patient admission. Multiple studies have examined this method of care, with encouraging results.[62–68]

In 2005, Shyu and colleagues[62] reported on a novel interdisciplinary intervention program for elderly patients with hip fracture. In a randomized trial, 137 patients with hip fracture were allocated to either an intervention group (n = 68) or a control group (n = 69). The intervention consisted of 3 routine interventions (in addition to orthopedic surgical services): geriatric (physician and nursing) consultation throughout admission, rehabilitation services (physiatrist, therapists, and geriatric nursing) beginning on postoperative day 1 and continuing after discharge (at home), and discharge planning by geriatric nursing services. The intervention group demonstrated improvements in recovering prefracture ambulatory capacity and ability to perform activities of daily living up to 3 months postoperatively, in comparison with the control group. Significant improvements were also demonstrated in range of motion (hip flexion), quadriceps strength, and measures of health-related quality of life. Most of these benefits were subsequently reported as being maintained at 1 year[63,69] and 2 years[70] following surgical repair.

A prospective, randomized trial of multidisciplinary comanagement of geriatric patients with hip fracture in Madrid, Spain was reported in 2005 by Vidan and colleagues.[64] All 319 elderly patients with hip fracture were admitted to the same orthopedic ward in a single hospital, received similar orthopedic care, and used the same hospital therapy and social work services. The intervention group (n = 155) was also assigned a geriatrician, rehabilitation specialist, and specialized social worker. The intervention group underwent comprehensive geriatric assessment, medical care by the geriatrician, therapy coordination by the rehabilitation specialist, and intensive social worker–mediated planning. Multidisciplinary meetings occurred within the first 72 hours of admission in the intervention group, and then weekly thereafter (while patients remained hospitalized). In the control group, specialist consultation was obtained only per orthopedic surgeon's direction when deemed to be indicated. Median length of stay trended shorter to 16 days in the intervention group from 18 days in the control group (P = .06). In-hospital mortality rates and medical complication rates decreased significantly in the intervention group (P = .03 and P = .003, respectively). Short-term (3 month) "partial recovery" of functional ambulation classification and of ability to perform activities of daily living were better in the intervention group (57%) than in the control group (44%, P = .03), but these differences disappeared at 6 and 12 months.

A hip-fracture service was developed at Johns Hopkins Bayview Medical Center in Baltimore, Maryland, and was reported on in 2005.[65] The development and details of the hip-fracture service were initially described in a concise letter to the editor of the *Journal of the American Geriatrics Society* in 2001.[71] In brief, elderly patients with hip fracture are admitted directly to the hip-fracture service. Preprinted emergency department, admission, and postoperative orders are used on all patients. Full cooperation between orthopedic surgery, anesthesiology, and medical services ensues. Discharge planning is initiated immediately, with a goal of discharge within 3 days in uncomplicated cases. The research report compared a total of 510 elderly patients with hip fracture treated before and after implementation of the hip-fracture service. The investigators demonstrated shorter hospital stays (5.7 vs 8.1 days), a higher rate of hip-fracture repair within 24 hours (63% vs 35%), and fewer medical complications (36% vs 51%) for patients admitted to the hip-fracture service in comparison with before its implementation.

Extensive investigation of multidisciplinary and protocol-driven comanagement of elderly patients with hip fracture has been accomplished at Highland Hospital (Rochester, NY).[60] Elderly patients with hip fracture are comanaged on a daily basis by a geriatrician and an orthopedic surgeon, with standardized care delivered to all patients in a protocol-driven fashion. The geriatric fracture center (GFC) at Highland Hospital was established in 2004. A cohort study comparing 193 patients with hip fracture treated at the GFC with 121 patients treated using standard care at a different hospital (administered by the same academic orthopedic department) was performed.[66] Although GFC patients with hip fracture tended to be older, had more medical comorbidities, and were more likely to reside in assisted living or total care institutions than the standard care group, they had shorter time to surgical treatment of hip fracture (24 vs 37 hours), fewer postoperative infections (2.3% vs 19.8%), and shorter length of stay (4.6 vs 8.3 days). Of note, restraint use was completely absent in the GFC group, whereas 14.1% of patients in the standard-care group required use of restraints during admission. Restraints are known to contribute to delirium in elderly hospitalized patients, especially those with mild preexisting dementia.[72] The investigators concluded that standardized care coupled with multidisciplinary comanagement resulted in improved outcomes and processes for elderly patients with hip fracture.

Based on early reported results, the Rochester model of geriatric fracture care appears to lead to improved clinical outcomes. However, it involves increased use of resources during the patient's admission. Increased use of resources entails added costs, although such increases in cost may be abrogated by shorter hospital stays and decreased rates of complication and readmission. An analysis of 193 elderly patients with hip fracture was performed by Kates and colleagues[68] to determine whether a profit or loss resulted from use of the GFC. Costs for the care of patients with hip fracture were compared with existing data within the New York State and United States databases. Through the use of the GFC program, the investigators were able to demonstrate costs

Table 4
Overview of cited studies based on 4 models of orthogeriatric care of hip fractures

Authors,[Ref.] Year	Model	Country	Inclusion Criteria	Exclusion Criteria	Study Design	LOS	Conclusion Summary	Level of Evidence
Kennie et al,[47] 1988	1	Great Britain	Elderly women with proximal femur fracture	Death before entering trial, pathologic fracture, discharge within 7 d of starting trial, unfit for transfer to peripheral hospital	Prospective, randomized	Control group 41 d, treatment group 24 d (95% CI for difference, 2–25 d)	Postoperative rehabilitation of benefit when provided in a location specializing in care of geriatric trauma patients	I
Naglie et al,[48] 2002	1	Canada	Hip-fracture surgery, ≥70 y old	In-hospital fracture, pathologic fracture, multiple trauma, prior surgery on ipsilateral hip, anticipated survival <6 mo, nursing home resident who requires personal assistance with ambulation, residence outside Toronto, ICU needed postoperatively, surgical failure	Prospective, randomized	Control group 20.9 d, treatment group 29.2 d (P<.001)	Postoperative interdisciplinary care did not result in improved outcomes	I
Swanson et al,[49] 1998	2	Australia	Hip fracture, ≥55 y old, independent mobility	Pathologic fracture, dementia, nursing home resident	Prospective, randomized	Control group 32.5 d, treatment group 21 d (P<.01)	LOS decreased with intervention	I
Zuckerman et al,[50] 1992	2	USA	Hip fracture, ≥65 y old, ambulatory	Pathologic fracture	Prospective, historical control	Control group 24.7 d, treatment group 23.2 d (NS)	Interdisciplinary care improves in-hospital care (less ICU, improved ambulation, fewer SNF admissions, fewer postoperative complications)	II

Study		Country	Inclusion Criteria	Exclusion Criteria	Study Design	LOS	Conclusion	Level
Koval et al,[6] 2004	2	USA	Hip fracture, ≥65 y old, independent living	Dementia	Prospective, historical control	Control group 21.6 d, treatment group 13 d ($P<.05$)	Decreased mortality, morbidity, LOS with intervention	II
Roberts et al,[51] 2004	2	Great Britain	Hip fracture, ≥65 y old	Multiple fractures, pathologic fracture	Prospective, cohort	Control group 37.2 d, treatment group 40.6 d (NS)	Intervention resulted in slightly longer LOS but improved mobility and reduced LTC admissions	II
Fisher et al,[52] 2006	2	Australia	Hip fracture, ≥60 y old	Pathologic fracture	Prospective, historical control	Control group 16.4 d, treatment group 15.9 d (NS)	Intervention reduced morbidity and mortality without effect on LOS	II
Cogan et al,[54] 2010	2	Ireland	Hip fracture, ≥65 y old	None	Retrospective, cohort	Control group 23.1 d, treatment group 30.3 d (P value not specified)	Intervention resulted in improvements in mortality and discharge destination	III
Khan et al,[53] 2002	2	Great Britain	Elderly hip-fracture patients	None	Prospective, historical control	Control group 26.1 d, treatment group 26.9 d (NS)	Intervention does not change outcomes	II
Boyd et al,[58] 1983	3	Great Britain	Elderly hip-fracture patients	None	Retrospective, cohort	Control group 66 d, treatment group 48 d ($P<.05$)	Intervention reduces LOS	III
Gilchrist et al,[55] 1988	3	Great Britain	Female, hip-fracture patients, ≥65 y old	Not transferred postoperatively to specific rehabilitation hospital	Prospective, randomized (methodological limitations)	Control group 47.7 d, treatment group 44 d (NS)	Intervention does not change LOS, mortality, or destination, but does identify more medical conditions	II
Adunsky et al,[57] 2003	3	Israel	Hip fracture, ≥65 y old, medically stable	Cannot actively rehabilitate, acute disability, fracture instability after surgery	Prospective, cohort	Control group 31.9 d, treatment group 26.9 d ($P<.01$)	Intervention resulted in improved outcomes	II
Adunsky et al,[59] 2005	3	Israel	Hip fracture, ≥60 y old	Admission to nonorthogeriatric ward postoperatively	Retrospective case series	29.9 d (no comparison group)	Orthogeriatric ward is practical and feasible	IV

(continued on next page)

Table 4
(continued)

Authors,[Ref.] Year	Model	Country	Inclusion Criteria	Exclusion Criteria	Study Design	LOS	Conclusion Summary	Level of Evidence
Stenvall et al,[56] 2007	3	Sweden	Hip fracture, ≥70 y old	Arthritis, pathologic fracture, nonambulatory, advanced renal disease	Prospective, randomized	Control group 40 d, treatment group 30 d ($P = .028$)	Intervention results in improvements in ADL performance and mobility	I
Shyu et al,[62] 2005	4	Taiwan	Hip fracture, ≥60 y old	Dementia, terminal illness	Prospective, randomized	Control group 10.23 d, treatment group 10.07 d (NS)	Intervention improves HRQOL, clinical outcomes, ability for self-care, and decreases depression	I
Vidan et al,[64] 2005	4	Spain	Hip fracture, ≥65 y old	Extreme dependency for ADLs, terminal illness, pathologic fracture	Prospective, randomized	Control group 18 d, treatment group 16 d (NS)	Intervention reduces in-hospital mortality and complications, early functional outcome is better	I
Khasraghi et al,[65] 2005	4	USA	Proximal femur fracture, ≥65 y old	Multiple fractures, pathologic fracture	Prospective, historical control	Control group 8.1 d, treatment group 5.7 d ($P<.05$)	Intervention reduces time to surgery from admission, LOS, and complications	II
Friedman et al,[66] 2009	4	USA	Proximal femur fracture, ≥60 y old	Pathologic fracture, major trauma, periprosthetic fracture, nonoperatively managed	Retrospective, cohort	Control group 8.3 d, treatment group 4.6 d ($P<.001$)	Intervention improves processes and outcomes	III
Kates et al,[68] 2011	4	USA	Hip fracture, ≥60 y old	Pathologic fracture, nonoperative management	Retrospective, cohort	Control group 6.3 d, treatment group 4.4 d (no *P* value provided)	Intervention reduces LOS, mortality, complication rates, readmission rates, and costs	III

Abbreviations: ADL, activities of daily living; CI, confidence interval; HRQOL, health-related quality of life; ICU, intensive care unit; LOS, length of stay; LTC, long-term care; NS, not significantly different; SNF, skilled nursing facility.

approximately 33% lower than expected costs, based on database extraction. Moreover, mortality rates, lengths of stay, readmission rates, and complication rates were all below national averages. These results indicate that protocol-driven multidisciplinary care for elderly patients with hip fractures leads to improved outcomes and decreased costs, despite an increase in resource use during patients' index admission.

Summary of Care Models

Of the 4 models of management of geriatric patients with hip fracture (**Table 4**), the final one described involves the most intricate collaboration between multiple services, and patients are "shared" completely between the geriatric and orthopedic services. The development of the geriatric fracture program at Highland Hospital did not occur overnight. It required an extended effort on the part of many different medical, surgical, and allied health services to arrive at a point where care of these patients would be seamless. This model, though the most attractive, may represent the most difficult one to implement. For hospitals considering clinical pathways for care of patients with hip fractures, perhaps beginning with model 2 (orthopedic admission with routine geriatric consultation) or model 3 (geriatric medicine admission with routine orthopedic consultation) would represent a good starting point, as they may be easier to implement. As all caregivers involved with managing patients with hip fractures become more accustomed to comanagement, a transition toward model 4 (true comanagement) could subsequently be considered.

What is required for a successful geriatric hip-fracture program? A team approach on the part of geriatricians and orthopedic surgeons seems reasonable. Hospitals that do not have subspecialty-trained geriatricians on staff may be able to substitute hospitalists; it is uncommon for most hospitals not to engage in the treatment of elderly patients. At the University of Missouri, not all primary care physicians involved with the hip-fracture protocol are subspecialty trained in geriatrics, yet the protocol has been proved successful by many measures (Della Rocca GJ, Moylan KC, Crist BD, Volgas DA, Stannard JP and Mehr DR, personal communication, 2012). A dedicated hospital unit, similar to the ACE unit developed at the Cleveland Clinic, and nurse coordinators may be beneficial for streamlining the care of geriatric patients with hip fracture. Ultimately, expenditures on the part of the hospital systems are required to get the program off the ground. Once established,

a well-run geriatric program will potentially save money for the hospital system.

SUMMARY

Care of the geriatric patient with a hip fracture is a complex endeavor. These patients present with multiple medical comorbidities and are often ill when they arrive at the emergency department with a fracture. Although expedited fracture care with surgery is beneficial in allowing for patient mobilization and a reduction of iatrogenic complications (such as pressure ulcers, pneumonia, and thromboembolic disease), the desire for rapid surgical care must be tempered by attention to medical optimization of the geriatric patient for surgery. Often this requires both time and the participation of multiple providers with different skill sets. Of the multiple existing models of geriatric hip-fracture care, those that involve both orthopedics and geriatric medicine on a comanagement basis appear to offer the benefit of shorter hospital stays, reduced morbidity and mortality rates (both in-hospital and short-term post discharge), and perhaps reduced costs. Although each patient requires individualized allocation of resources, these models represent methods for streamlined delivery of care that lends attention to each of a given patient's problems. Expedited surgical care of the elderly patient with a hip fracture, accomplished in the setting of multidisciplinary preoperative and postoperative care, appears to yield improved outcomes for this subset of frail patients.

With more and more centers describing varying degrees of success through the use of comanagement protocols for elderly patients with hip fracture, a logical next step may entail an expansion of hip-fracture protocols to all elderly patients with fractures. Other fragility fractures are known to occur in the frail elderly (distal radius fractures, vertebral compression fractures), as are other fractures not commonly classified as fractures of fragility (proximal humerus fractures, distal femur fractures, sacral insufficiency fractures). Elderly patients with these fractures may have accompanying comorbid conditions that are very similar to those that accompany hip fracture. Perhaps inclusion of mechanisms for screening and initiation of treatment for osteoporosis should also be incorporated in geriatric fracture programs. The fracture may represent the sentinel event that mobilizes orthopedic, geriatric, and osteoporosis management, resulting in improved quality of life and decreased mortality in the frail elderly population after fracture repair.

REFERENCES

1. Youm T, Koval KJ, Zuckerman JD. The economic impact of geriatric hip fractures. Am J Orthop 1999;28:423–8.
2. Cooper C, Campion G, Meltion LJ. Hip fractures in the elderly: a worldwide projection. Osteoporos Int 1992;2:285–9.
3. Cummings SR, Rubin SM, Black D. The future of hip fractures in the United States: numbers, costs, and potential effects of post-menopausal estrogen. Clin Orthop Relat Res 1990;252:163–6.
4. Haentjens P, Autier P, Barette M, et al. The economic cost of hip fractures among elderly women: a one-year, prospective, observational cohort study with matched-pair analysis. J Bone Joint Surg Am 2001;83:493–500.
5. Wiktorowicz ME, Goeree R, Papaioannou A, et al. Economic implications of hip fracture: health service use, institutional care and cost in Canada. Osteoporos Int 2001;12:271–8.
6. Koval KJ, Chen AL, Aharonoff GB, et al. Clinical pathway for hip fractures in the elderly—the Hospital for Joint Diseases experience. Clin Orthop Relat Res 2004;425:72–81.
7. Zuckerman JD, Skovron ML, Koval KJ, et al. Postoperative complications and mortality associated with operative delay in older patients who have a fracture of the hip. J Bone Joint Surg Am 1995;77:1551–6.
8. Hamlet WP, Lieberman JR, Freedman EL, et al. Influence of health status and the timing of surgery on mortality in hip fracture patients. Am J Orthop 1997;26:621–7.
9. Doruk H, Mas MR, Yildiz C, et al. The effect of the timing of hip fracture surgery on the activity of daily living and mortality in elderly. Arch Gerontol Geriatr 2004;39:179–85.
10. Orosz GM, Magaziner J, Hannan EL, et al. Association of timing of surgery for hip fracture and patient outcomes. JAMA 2004;291:1738–43.
11. Gdalevich M, Cohen D, Yosef D, et al. Morbidity and mortality after hip fracture: the impact of operative delay. Arch Orthop Trauma Surg 2004;124:334–40.
12. Moran CG, Wenn RT, Sikand M, et al. Early mortality after hip fracture: is delay before surgery important? J Bone Joint Surg Am 2005;87:483–9.
13. McGuire KJ, Bernstein J, Polsky D, et al. The 2004 Marshall Urist award: delays until surgery after hip fracture increases mortality. Clin Orthop Relat Res 2004;428:294–301.
14. Jyrkka J, Enlund H, Korhonen MJ, et al. Polypharmacy status as an indicator of mortality in an elderly population. Drugs Aging 2009;26:1039–48.
15. Devas M. Geriatric orthopaedics. London: Academic Press; 1977.
16. Hempsall VJ, Robertson DR, Campbell MJ, et al. Orthopaedic geriatric care: is it effective? A prospective population-based comparison of outcome in fractured neck of femur. J R Coll Physicians Lond 1990;24:47–50.
17. Elliot JR, Wilkinson TJ, Hanger HC, et al. The added effectiveness of early geriatrician involvement on acute orthopaedic wards to orthogeriatric rehabilitation. N Z Med J 1996;109:72–3.
18. World Health Organization. Assessment of fracture risk and its application to screening for postmenopausal osteoporosis: report of a WHO study group. World Health Organ Tech Rep Ser 1994; 843:1–129.
19. Penrod JD, Litke A, Hawkes WG, et al. Heterogeneity in hip fracture patients: age, functional status, and comorbidity. J Am Geriatr Soc 2007;55:407–13.
20. Baranzini F, Diurni M, Ceccon F, et al. Fall-related injuries in a nursing home setting: is polypharmacy a risk factor? BMC Health Serv Res 2009;9:228.
21. Coutinho ES, Fletcher A, Bloch KV, et al. Risk factors for falls with severe fracture in elderly people living in a middle-income country: a case control study. BMC Geriatr 2008;8:21.
22. Lyons LJ, Nevins MA. Non-treatment of hip fractures in senile patients. JAMA 1977;238:1175–6.
23. Niemann KM, Mankin HJ. Fractures about the hip in an institutionalized patient population: II. Survival and ability to walk again. J Bone Joint Surg Am 1968;50:1327–40.
24. Sherk HH, Snape WJ, Loprete FL. Internal fixation versus nontreatment of hip fractures in senile patients. Clin Orthop Relat Res 1979;141:196–8.
25. Kenzora JE, McCarthy RE, Lowell JD, et al. Hip fracture mortality: relation to age, treatment, preoperative illness, time of surgery, and complications. Clin Orthop Relat Res 1984;186:45–56.
26. Sexson SB, Lehner JT. Factors affecting hip fracture mortality. J Orthop Trauma 1987;1:298–305.
27. White BL, Fisher WD, Laurin CA. Rate of mortality for elderly patients after fracture of the hip in the 1980's. J Bone Joint Surg Am 1987;69:1335–40.
28. Davis TR, Sher JL, Porter BB, et al. The timing of surgery for intertrochanteric femoral fractures. Injury 1988;19:244–6.
29. Davidson TI, Bodey WN. Factors influencing survival following fractures of the upper end of the femur. Injury 1986;17:12–4.
30. Ricci WM, Della Rocca GJ, Combs C, et al. The medical and economic impact of preoperative cardiac testing in elderly patients with hip fractures. Injury 2007;38(Suppl 3):S49–52.
31. Grimes JP, Gregory PM, Noveck H, et al. The effects of time-to-surgery on mortality and morbidity in patients following hip fracture. Am J Med 2002; 112:702–9.
32. Devas MB. Geriatric orthopaedics. Br Med J 1974; 1(5900):190–2.
33. Department of Health (Great Britain). The new NHS: modern, dependable. London: HMSO; 1997.

34. Healy WL, Ayers ME, Iorio R, et al. Impact of a clinical pathway and implant standardization on total hip arthroplasty: a clinical and economic study of short-term patient outcome. J Arthroplasty 1998; 13:266–76.

35. Cannon CP, Jand MH, Barh R, et al. Critical pathways for management of patients with acute coronary syndromes: an assessment by the National Heart Attack Alert Program. Am Heart J 2002;143: 777–89.

36. Browne GJ, McCaskill ME, Fasher BJ, et al. The benefits of using clinical pathways for managing acute paediatric illness in an emergency department. J Qual Clin Pract 2001;21:50–5.

37. Sweeney AB, Flora HS, Chaloner EJ, et al. Integrated care pathways for vascular surgery: an analysis of the first 18 months. Postgrad Med J 2002;78: 175–7.

38. Ogilvie-Harris DJ, Botsford DJ, Hawker RW. Elderly patients with hip fractures: improved outcome with the use of care maps with high-quality medical and nursing protocols. J Orthop Trauma 1993;7: 428–37.

39. Tallis G, Balla JI. Critical path analysis for the management of fractured neck of femur. Aust J Public Health 1995;19:155–9.

40. Choong PF, Langford AK, Dowsey MM, et al. Clinical pathway for fractured neck of femur: a prospective, controlled study. Med J Aust 2000;172: 423–7.

41. Santamaria N, Houghton L, Kimmel L, et al. Clinical pathways for fractured neck of femur: a cohort study of health related quality of life, patient satisfaction and clinical outcome. Aust J Adv Nurs 2003;20(3): 24–9.

42. March LM, Cameron ID, Cumming RG, et al. Mortality and morbidity after hip fracture: can evidence based clinical pathways make a difference? J Rheumatol 2000;27:2227–31.

43. New Zealand Guidelines Group. The management of hip fracture in adults. Wellington (New Zealand): New Zealand Guidelines Group; 2011.

44. Chevalley T, Hoffmeyer P, Bonjour JP, et al. An osteoporosis clinical pathway for the medical management of patients with low-trauma fracture. Osteoporos Int 2002;13:450–5.

45. Pioli G, Giusti A, Barone A. Orthogeriatric care for the elderly with hip fractures: where are we? Aging Clin Exp Res 2008;20:113–22.

46. Kammerlander C, Roth T, Friedman SM, et al. Orthogeriatric service—a literature review comparing different models. Osteoporos Int 2010;21(Suppl 4): S637–46.

47. Kennie DC, Reid J, Richardson IR, et al. Effectiveness of geriatric rehabilitative care after fractures of the proximal femur in elderly women: a randomised clinical trial. BMJ 1988;297:1083–6.

48. Naglie G, Tansey C, Kirkland JL, et al. Interdisciplinary inpatient care for elderly people with hip fracture: a randomized controlled trial. Can Med Assoc J 2002;167:25–32.

49. Swanson CE, Day GA, Yelland CE, et al. The management of elderly patients with femoral fractures: a randomised controlled trial of early intervention versus standard care. Med J Aust 1998;169: 515–8.

50. Zuckerman JD, Sakales SR, Fabian DR, et al. Hip fractures in geriatric patients: results of an interdisciplinary hospital care program. Clin Orthop Relat Res 1992;274:213–25.

51. Roberts HC, Pickering RM, Onslow E, et al. The effectiveness of implementing a care pathway for femoral neck fracture in older people: a prospective controlled before and after study. Age Ageing 2004; 22:178–84.

52. Fisher AA, Davis MW, Rubenach SE, et al. Outcomes for older patients with hip fractures: the impact of orthopedic and geriatric medicine cocare. J Orthop Trauma 2006;20:172–8.

53. Khan R, Fernandez C, Hashifl F, et al. Combined orthogeriatric care in the management of hip fractures: a prospective study. Ann R Coll Surg Engl 2002;84: 122–4.

54. Cogan L, Martin AJ, Kelly LA, et al. An audit of hip fracture services in the Mater Hospital Dublin 2001 compared with 2006. Ir J Med Sci 2010; 179:51–5.

55. Gilchrist WJ, Newman RJ, Hamblen DL, et al. Prospective randomised study of an orthopaedic geriatric inpatient service. BMJ 1988;297:1116–8.

56. Stenvall M, Olofsson B, Nyberg L, et al. Improved performance in activities of daily living and mobility after a multidisciplinary postoperative rehabilitation in older people with femoral neck fracture: a randomized controlled trial with 1-year follow-up. J Rehabil Med 2007;39:232–8.

57. Adunsky A, Lusky A, Arad M, et al. A comparative study of rehabilitation outcomes of elderly hip fracture patients: the advantage of a comprehensive orthogeriatric approach. J Gerontol A Biol Sci Med Sci 2003;58:542–7.

58. Boyd RV, Hawthorne J, Wallace WA, et al. The Nottingham orthogeriatric unit after 1000 admissions. Injury 1983;15:193–6.

59. Adunsky A, Arad M, Levi R, et al. Five-year experience with the 'Sheba' model of comprehensive orthogeriatric care for elderly hip fracture patients. Disabil Rehabil 2005;27:1123–7.

60. Friedman SM, Mendelson DA, Kates SL, et al. Geriatric co-management of proximal femur fractures: total quality management and protocol-driven care result in better outcomes for a frail patient population. J Am Geriatr Soc 2008;56: 1349–56.

61. Covinsky KE, Palmer RM, Kresevic DM, et al. Improving functional outcomes in older patients: lessons from an acute care for elders unit. Jt Comm J Qual Improv 1998;24:63–76.

62. Shyu YI, Liang J, Wu CC, et al. A pilot investigation of the short-term effects of an interdisciplinary intervention program on elderly patients with hip fracture in Taiwan. J Am Geriatr Soc 2005;53: 811–8.

63. Shyu YI, Liang J, Wu CC, et al. Interdisciplinary intervention for hip fracture in older Taiwanese: benefits last for 1 year. J Gerontol A Biol Sci Med Sci 2008; 63:92–7.

64. Vidan M, Serra JA, Moreno C, et al. Efficacy of a comprehensive geriatric intervention in older patients hospitalized for hip fracture: a randomized, controlled trial. J Am Geriatr Soc 2005;53:1476–82.

65. Khasraghi FA, Christmas C, Lee EJ, et al. Effectiveness of a multidisciplinary team approach to hip fracture management. J Surg Orthop Adv 2005;14: 27–31.

66. Friedman SM, Mendelson DA, Bingham KW, et al. Impact of a comanaged geriatric fracture center on short-term hip fracture outcomes. Arch Intern Med 2009;169:1712–7.

67. Kates SL, Mendelson DA, Friedman SM. Co-managed care for fragility hip fractures (Rochester model). Osteoporos Int 2010;21(Suppl 4):S621–5.

68. Kates SL, Mendelson DA, Friedman SM. The value of an organized fracture program for the elderly: early results. J Orthop Trauma 2011;25:233–7.

69. Shyu YI, Liang J, Wu CC, et al. An interdisciplinary intervention for older Taiwanese patients after surgery for hip fracture improves health-related quality of life. BMC Musculoskelet Disord 2010;11: 225.

70. Shyu YI, Liang J, Wu CC, et al. Two-year effects of interdisciplinary intervention for hip fracture in older Taiwanese. J Am Geriatr Soc 2010;58:1081–9.

71. De Jonge KE, Christmas C, Andersen R, et al. Hip fracture service—an interdisciplinary model of care. J Am Geriatr Soc 2001;49:1737–8.

72. McCusker J, Cole M, Abrahamowicz M, et al. Environmental risk factors for delirium in hospitalized older people. J Am Geriatr Soc 2001;49: 1327–34.

Biomechanical Considerations for Surgical Stabilization of Osteoporotic Fractures

Ljiljana Bogunovic, MD, Steven M. Cherney, MD,
Marcus A. Rothermich, MD, Michael J. Gardner, MD*

KEYWORDS

- Osteoporotic fracture • Fragility fracture • Locked plating • Cephalomedullary nail
- Intertrochanteric fracture • Proximal humerus fracture • Distal femur fracture

KEY POINTS

- The incidence of osteoporotic fractures is steadily increasing.
- Diminished bone mass and frequent comminution make fixation of osteoporotic fractures difficult.
- Locked plating enhances fixation stability in osteoporotic bone.
- Adequate fixation of unstable intertrochanteric fractures requires fixation with intramedullary device.

INTRODUCTION

Osteoporosis is a common disorder of the elderly, affecting nearly 8 million women and 2 million men in the United States alone.[1] Driven by an imbalance in bone turnover, osteoporosis is characterized by decreased bone mass and altered bone microstructural properties. An increase in osteoclast activity combined with a decrease in osteoblast activity leads to overall bone mineral loss. Metaphyseal skeletal regions with a high proportion of cancellous bone are affected most severely. A diagnosis of osteoporosis is often heralded by the occurrence of a fragility fracture; common sites include the distal radius, proximal femur, distal femur, and proximal humerus. Each year, an estimated 1.5 million US adults sustain a fracture after a low-energy injury, such as a fall from standing height. The associated morbidity, mortality, and medical costs are significant. The 1-year mortality of elderly hip fractures has been reported to be as high as 30%,[2] and the overall cost of osteoporotic fracture medical treatment is an estimated $18 billion a year.[1]

EFFECT OF OSTEOPOROSIS ON FRACTURE FIXATION

Bone failure, not implant failure, defines the challenge of osteoporotic fracture fixation. Disease-driven alterations in structural bone properties substantially weaken implant fixation in osteoporotic bone, particularly when nonlocking screws are used. Multiple biomechanical studies have demonstrated an association between bone density and screw fixation strength. As bone mass decreases, so does the holding power of a screw.[3] Screw and implant cutout are common modes of failure in osteoporotic bone. This situation is magnified in metaphyseal bone where the trabecular network of cancellous bone is especially affected by osteoporotic changes. An additional factor complicating overall success of osteoporotic fracture fixation is an increased frequency

Funding Sources: Dr Gardner: None.
Conflict of Interest: Dr Gardner: Consultant: Synthes, Stryker, RTI Biologics, and DGIMed Ortho.
Department of Orthopedic Surgery, Washington University, 660 South Euclid Avenue, St Louis, MO 63110-1010, USA
* Corresponding author.
E-mail address: gardnerm@wudosis.wustl.edu

Orthop Clin N Am 44 (2013) 183–200
http://dx.doi.org/10.1016/j.ocl.2013.01.006
0030-5898/13/$ – see front matter © 2013 Elsevier Inc. All rights reserved.

of fracture comminution in the setting of decreased bone mass. Despite that healing potential is unaltered in osteoporotic bone, impaired fixation increases the risk of reduction loss, malunion, and nonunion. Given these challenges, implant modification and novel designs have been developed in an effort to improve fixation in osteoporotic bone.

FIXATION: GENERAL CONSIDERATIONS
Screws

Screws are one of the most common implant types used in fracture fixation. Whether used in isolation for interfragmentary fixation or in combination with a plate, conventional screw fixation is dependent on the force generated between screw threads and the bone. Two basic screw designs exist, cortical and cancellous. For both types, screw purchase is reliant on thread engagement in bone tissue and highly dependent bone mineral density. Cortical screws are characterized by smaller thread diameter, a smaller pitch, and a shallower thread and are designed for placement in more dense cortical bone. As a general rule, screw fixation should be placed in cortical bone whenever possible to optimize purchase. The cancellous screw is a simple modification of screw design created to address reduced fixation strength in less-dense metaphyseal or osteoporotic bone. An increase in screw thread diameter and pitch provide more surface area for bone purchase. Once bone mineral density falls below 0.4 g/cm^3, however, changes in screw geometry can no longer improve fixation strength.[4]

Augmentation

Bone augments, including polymethylmethacrylate and tricalcium phosphate bone cement, have been used to increase screw purchase in weaker osteoporotic bone. Cement can be injected into porous regions of metaphyseal bone and left to harden. The drying cement interdigitates with the bone trabeculae, increasing the overall material density and thereby improving subsequent screw purchase. More localized cement application is achieved by direct injection of cement into newly drilled screw holes.[5] After filling with cement, screws are inserted into the holes but not tightened until the cement has hardened. Cement augmentation has been suggested to improve screw pullout strength in osteoporotic bone.[6] The majority of biomechanical testing of cement augmentation, however, has involved pullout testing of screw strength rather than functional loading, the latter of which is more representative of a clinical setting. A disadvantage of polymethylmethacrylate is that

it does not reabsorb and becomes permanent, making it difficult to remove if the need arises. In addition, the exothermic curing process of cement may induce thermonecrosis to adjacent bone and compromise fracture healing. For these reasons, the authors do not advocate routine use of polymethylmethacrylate augmentation. An advantage of alternative bone augments, such as tricalcium phosphate cement, is that it is resorbable and osteoconductive. The tricalcium phosphate cement provides a scaffold for bone progenitor cells and over time is remodeled to a patient's native osteoporotic bone. With both cement types, care must be taken to avoid placement directly into the fracture site, because this may impair healing between fragments.

Screws coated with hydroxyapatite or bisphosphonates have also been designed as a means of improving implant fixation.[7] Hydroxyapatite functions to improve initial screw purchase, whereas the bisphosphonate coating promotes the development of increased bone mass at the screw-bone interface.[8] Both materials have been shown in biomechanical cadaver and animal studies to improve screw fixation; however, augmentation using bisphosphonate coating takes time for the beneficial effects to occur (approximately 2 weeks).[9]

Traditional Plates

Traditional plate fixation achieves fracture stability through creation of preload and friction force between the plate and bone, and it is, therefore, classified as a load-bearing device. In managing osteoporotic fractures, several principles can help to achieve success. In general, bridge plating of osteoporotic fractures should be done with caution, because it relies solely on the implant for stability without intrinsic bone contact, but with long comminuted segments is acceptable and can be successful. With increasing fracture gap, the strain across the implant grows, predisposing the construct to failure. The best way unload strain on the plate construct is to achieve cortical contact at the fracture site and, in the setting of comminution, this may require shortening of the bone. Shortening alters anatomy, however, and predictably creates a malunion, so intentional fracture shortening should be done with careful consideration. Thoughtful screw position is critical to creation of a successful construct. The working length of the plate, defined as the distance between the closest screws on either side of the fracture, is the most important determinant of the axial and torsional stiffness. In order to optimize stiffness and bending rigidity, screws should be positioned as close to the fracture as possible, while avoiding comminution. Longer plates have been shown to significantly improve bending strength.[10] As described in a study by Sanders and colleagues,[10] 8-hole and 10-hole plates with screw placement near the fracture site demonstrated improved biomechanical properties compared with a 6-hole plate with screws placed in every hole. The ideal plate construct minimizes working length and maximizes plate length, whereas the addition of intervening screws does little to improve fixation strength. Finally, surgeons should not underestimate the utility of buttress/antiglide plate fixation of osteoporotic fractures. Successful fracture alignment and stability can be achieved, even in osteoporotic bone, with placement of an antiglide plate in areas subject to shear force, such as the lateral malleolus and the proximal tibia. A properly positioned antiglide plate inherently prevents fracture displacement and minimizes the reliance on screw fixation.[11]

Locking Plates

Plate design has evolved over the past decade to address difficulties associated with osteoporotic fracture fixation. The development of locked plating revolutionized fracture fixation in weaker bone, by shifting the focus of fracture stability to the screw/plate interface rather than relying on friction generated by a screw compressing plate to bone.[12] Locked plating offers angular stability, with each screw becoming a fixed-angle device within the plate. Angular stability serves to minimize screw displacement under bending loads, because locking prevents screw toggle within the plate. Also, failure of locking plates requires failure of the entire screw plate construct, which differs significantly from traditional plating, where failure can result from loosening or cutout of a single poorly fixed screw. The biomechanical benefits of locked plating are especially helpful in weaker metaphyseal bone and osteoporotic diaphyseal bone. Locked plating, however, has not demonstrated an advantage over traditional plating in diaphyseal bone.[13]

Challenges of Locking Plates in Osteoporotic Bone

Recent data have shown that the stiffness achieved with locked plating may be too high for certain osteoporotic fractures, stimulating modifications of locked plating technique. The fixed-angle design of locked screws results in increased stress at the screw-bone interface because there is no load transfer between the plate and bone

surface, as seen in traditional plating. The high stiffness of the plate construct, relative to the low stiffness of osteoporotic bone, generates a stress-riser effect, predisposing the construct to periprosthetic fracture, especially under bending loads. The incidence of secondary periprosthetic fracture after locked plating has been reported to be as high as 2.6%.[14] Replacement of the outermost locked screws with traditional screws has been shown to improve bending strength by 40% without affecting the ability of the plate to withstand torsional or compressive loads.[15]

The increased stiffness that characterizes locked plates has also been implicated in fracture nonunion. Fixed-angle stability makes locked plating an attractive option in the treatment of comminuted fractures. Fixation of comminuted fractures, however, especially those in periarticular regions, relies on micromotion between fracture fragments and secondary healing through callus formation. Rigid locked fixation may eliminate this micromotion and contribute to a high nonunion rate of up to 19% in fractures, such as the distal femur.[16] Several methods have been described to decrease stiffness and enhance interfragmentary micromotion in locked plate constructs. The technique of far cortical locking reduces construct stiffness without compromising strength. The midshaft of far cortical locking screws is modified such that the screws lock into the far cortex and the plate but bypass the near cortex. The increased working length of the screw results in a reduction in stiffness and allows for parallel interfragmentary motion at the near cortex, which promotes callus formation and fracture healing.[17] Furthermore, far cortical locking constructs display a biphasic stiffness behavior. Under smaller loads, stiffness of the construct is low, but stiffness gradually increases with progressively higher loads. At high loads, far cortical locking results in a construct that is 54% stronger in torsion, 21% stronger in bending, and 84% as strong under compression compared with standard locked plating.[17] This technique can be applied to periarticular fractures, where far cortical locking screws are placed in the diaphyseal segment and standard locking screws are used in the metaphyseal and periarticular portions, which lack a far cortex.[18] An alternative to far cortical locking is the use of near cortical slots. The use of slotted holes at the near cortex in place of standard holes functions similarly to the far cortical locking technique in that construct stiffness is reduced while overall fixation stability is maintained.[19–21] The cost with these newer technologies is much greater than conventional implants, and similar stiffness effects may be obtained with cortical screw fixation in the diaphyseal segment.

An additional disadvantage of pure locked plating is the inability of the plate-screw construct to facilitate reduction. Although compression generated between a traditional screw and plate can be used to affect fracture reduction, the insertion of a fixed-angle screw does not reduce a fracture. When using pure locked plating construct, surgeons must reduce the fracture before fixation. The advent of hybrid plates combines the advantages of traditional and locked plating. Hybrid plates contain holes, which accommodate both traditional and locked screws. The sequence of fracture fixation with hybrid plates proceeds as follows: the bone is reduced to the plate using a traditional screw and then locking screws are placed to improve construct strength and protect the cortical screws. Despite initial concerns about construct stability, the addition of non-locked screws results in minimal reduction in axial strength, improved torsional strength, and equivalent bending strength compared with fully locked plates.[22] When using a hybrid technique in osteoporotic diaphyseal bone, a minimum of 3 bicortical locking screws should be inserted on either of the fracture to optimized torsional stiffness.[23] Locking screws placed on either end of nonlocked screws has also been suggested as having a protected effect and minimizing construct fatigability.[23]

Intramedullary Nails

Intramedullary nails (IMNs) are another common implant choice and the gold standard for diaphyseal fractures of the tibia and femur. IMNs are load-sharing devices and less susceptible to implant failure compared with plate fixation. The central location of the nail within the medullary canal distributes load equally across the construct, in contrast to plate fixation in which stress is eccentrically focused on the implant side of the cortex. Insertion of the nail proximal or distal to the fracture site allows for preservation of the surrounding soft tissue, periosteum, and fracture hematoma, further promoting healing. In treating osteoporotic patients, wide-diameter nails may be required to accommodate the expansion of the medullary canal seen in osteoporosis. Fracture fixation with an IMN generally allows for early weight bearing, a useful advantage in elderly patients where immobility is associated with increased morbidity.

Fracture fixation with an IMN requires placement of interlocking screws to achieve control of axial and rotational displacement. The weakness of IMN fixation, especially in osteoporotic bone, is the strength of interlocking screw fixation at the metaphysis. The same challenges of screw purchase in weak bone seen with plates arise here as well. Alternations to distal interlocks may be necessary to achieve adequate fixation in weaker bone. Placement of interlock screws in multiple planes has been shown to enhance fixation, as has cement augmentation or use of a washer.[24] Other newer designs offer a blade-like device as an interlock and fixed-angle interlocking screws.[25]

Osteoporotic fracture fixation is challenging and often requires different techniques and implants to maximize fixation. With the availability of locking screws and locking periarticular plates, screw augmentation with cement is not commonly used. In the diaphyseal segment of osteoporotic fractures, locking screws can improve fixation strength, whether used exclusively or in combination with cortical screws (hybrid fixation). For metaphyseal osteoporotic fractures, nails provide some advantages, but locking plates may facilitate reduction and provide more fixation points in the short end segment and should be considered strongly.

PROXIMAL HUMERUS
Introduction

Fractures of the proximal humerus are some of the most common types of fragility fractures. More than 184,000 emergency room visits in 2008 were for proximal humerus fractures and it is projected that, by 2030, 275,000 proximal humerus fractures will be seen in emergency departments each year. The fracture rates per 100,000 individuals increase exponentially as age increases and are particularly pronounced in women. Despite the increasing burden of proximal humerus fractures, most do not require operative treatment. Nondisplaced fractures represent up to 85% of all proximal humerus fractures,[26] the majority of which can be successfully treated nonoperatively. At some centers, however, referrals increase the incidence of displaced 2-part, 3-part, and 4-part fractures and may compromise up to 53% of all proximal humerus fractures that are seen.[27]

Despite the high percentage of nondisplaced and stable fractures, some patients with displaced and unstable fractures benefit from operative fixation to restore anatomy and allow early rehabilitation. Operative fixation of osteoporotic proximal humerus fracture is challenging and is related to the anatomy of the proximal humerus in osteoporotic patients, specifically the small tuberosity fragments, the poor bone quality, and the inability to place bicortical screws into the humeral head.

The proximal humeral head, in particular the central portion, and humeral metaphysis are common areas of resorption during osteoporosis. The humeral head has even been described as similar to an eggshell or a grapefruit, which helps understand how the quality of bone, coupled with the inability to place bicortical fixation in the humeral head, limits a surgeon's ability to obtain and maintain secure fixation. In addition to osteoporosis, avascular necrosis is another consideration when treating osteoporotic proximal humerus fractures and is a result of the traumatic and surgical insult to the tenuous blood supply to the humeral head. The posterior humeral circumflex artery tends to be the dominant arterial supply to the humeral head.[28] This blood supply is damaged at the time of injury in approximately 80% patients; however, neovascularization is believed to occur with preservation of perfusion observed even in 3 and 4 part fractures.[29,30] With proper surgical technique and careful attention to avoid unnecessary soft tissue stripping, avascular necrosis is a rare complication, with necrosis occurring in 2.3% to 3.1% of patients in 2 recent case series.[29,31]

Surgical Techniques

Closed reduction and percutaneous pinning

Closed reduction and percutaneous pinning can be a viable surgical option; however, the indications for this technique are narrow. Fractures must not extend below the surgical neck, the fracture must be minimally comminuted, and the fracture must be able to be reduced and stabilized in a closed or minimally open fashion. The advantages of this procedure are that minimal soft tissue stripping may lead to less avascular necrosis and increased postoperative range of motion.[32] Intermediate outcomes for patients treated with closed reduction and percutaneous pinning have revealed that osteonecrosis is a late occurrence, as far as 8 years after initial intervention. Overall, the need for revision surgery is not increased despite the increased incidence of late osteonecrosis.[33]

Intramedullary nail

Recent development of specialized IMNs has led to an increased interest in using locked nails as an alternative to open reduction and internal fixation (ORIF) with locking plates. IMNs, in theory, involve less soft tissue stripping and offer the advantage of a load-sharing device.[34] IMNs can be used to treat 2-part, 3-part, and 4-part fracture patterns but are best suited to 2-part fractures.[35,36] Meticulous surgical technique must be used to preserve and repair the supraspinatus tendon and to avoid nail prominence. A recent

randomized controlled trial demonstrated that at 3-year follow-up, outcomes between the IMN and locking plate groups were similar for American Shoulder and Elbow Surgeons score, pain, and supraspinatus strength. In this trial, the locked nail had significantly shorter operative times and less blood loss (**Fig. 1**).[35]

Locking plates

Specialized locking plates designed for the proximal humerus allow for ORIF of proximal humerus fractures. The specialized designs allow for multiple locking screws to be placed into the humeral head, which help decrease the risk of screw pullout and varus collapse. Certain plate designs also now incorporate holes for sutures, which can be used to augment repairs, particularly for tuberosity fragments and comminuted fracture patterns.[37] Care must be taken to avoid superior placement of the plate, which causes impingement with shoulder abduction. Furthermore, there is a risk of screw penetration into the articular surface as the surgeon attempts to obtain good screw purchase in the dense subchondral bone. Restoration of the medial calcar and proper placement of an inferomedial oblique screw in the humeral head is thought to increase the likelihood of maintaining fracture reduction.[38] Additionally, structural augmentation with either calcium phosphate cement[39] or a fibular strut allograft may substantially reduce the risk of reduction loss and implant failure (**Fig. 2**).[40,41]

Shoulder arthroplasty

Shoulder arthroplasty was once recommended as the primary treatment of 3-part and 4-part fractures; however, this has fallen out of favor in a majority of these fracture patterns.[42] As site-specific locking plates have been developed, the concern for avascular necrosis and nonunion has decreased. Furthermore, nonunion or malunion of tuberosity fragments have been shown to correlate with poor outcomes.[43] For these reasons, shoulder arthroplasty has become a salvage procedure in most cases. Primary arthroplasty still may be the best surgical option in the face of multifragmentary head cleavage or early avascularity of the head fragments (**Fig. 3**).[34]

Clinical Outcomes and Complications

Patient outcomes after fixation of osteoporotic proximal humerus fractures are generally good but can vary with patient age and fracture pattern. Advanced age and more complicated fracture types are associated with worse outcomes.[44–47] Patients should be counseled that their functional outcomes are likely to continue to improve over

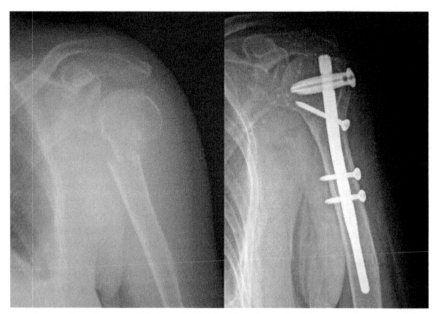

Fig. 1. Osteoporotic proximal humerus fracture (*left*). Fixation of proximal humerus fracture with a locked intramedullary nail (IMN) (*right*). (*From* Zhu Y, Lu Y, Shen J, et al. Locking intramedullary nails and locking plates in the treatment of two-part proximal humeral surgical neck fractures: a prospective randomized trial with a minimum of three years of follow-up. J Bone Joint Surg Am 2011;93:159; with permission.)

a long period of time and that their outcome is also greatly influenced by postinjury or postoperative rehabilitation.[47,48]

Successful outcome can be achieved with multiple techniques. ORIF with a locked plating remains a reliable method for unstable 2-part,

3-part, and 4-part fractures.[45] Postoperative Constant scores of an average of 70 can be achieved at 1 year.[49,50] Complications include osteonecrosis, screw perforation of the humeral head, and loss of fixation.[45,46,50] Locked IMN fixation is another option, best used in patients with 2-part

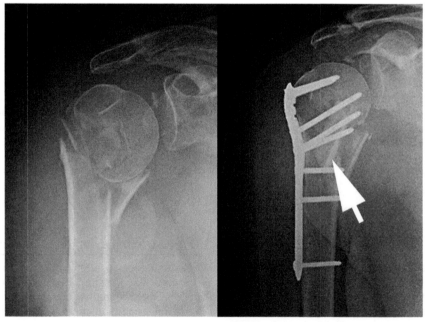

Fig. 2. Case example of a 73-year-old woman with a varus unstable proximal humerus fracture with medial calcar comminution (*left*). Given her high risk of fixation failure with traditional ORIF techniques, a fibular strut allograft was used to reconstruct the medial calcar region (*arrow*) (*right*).

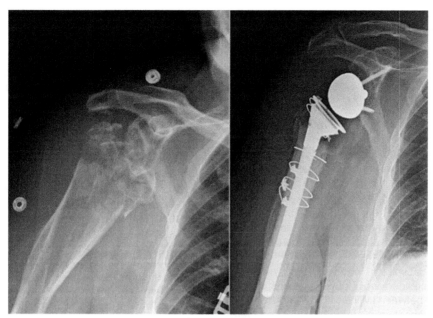

Fig. 3. Comminuted proximal humerus fracture in a 79-year-old man (*left*) treated with reverse total shoulder arthroplasty (*right*).

fractures involving the surgical neck.[51] Lower complication rates (4% vs 31%) have been reported with IMNs compared with locked plate fixation of similar fracture patterns.[35]

Given the high frequency of poor quality bone, closed reduction and percutaneous pinning are not often used in the treatment of the majority of osteoporotic proximal humerus fractures. Finally, hemiarthroplasty is indicated in those fractures not amenable to fixation, such as fractures with significant comminution or with head splitting patterns. Hemiarthroplasty has been shown effective in alleviating pain, but unpredictable limitations in range of motion have been reported in some patients postoperatively, worsening patient-rated outcome.[52] Tuberosity displacement or nonunion is a worrisome complication of shoulder hemiarthroplasty.

HUMERAL SHAFT
Introduction

Fractures of the humeral shaft have an incidence of 3% to 5%, account for more than 57,000 emergency department visits annually in the United States, and tend to occur in a bimodal age distribution.[53] The first peak is in young men and the second peak in elderly female patients.[54] Fractures occurring in patients older than 50 years of age account for 60% of the total humeral diaphyseal fractures observed and represent a true fragility fracture.

Most humeral shaft fractures can be treated nonoperatively. Functional bracing, first described by Sarmiento and colleagues,[55] expect to have successful outcomes in 90% of cases. Furthermore, 98% of closed injuries and 94% of open injuries go on to clinical union with conservative treatment. Malunion (greater than 16° of angulation in any plane) occurs with greater frequency in nonoperatively treated fractures, resulting in combined varus and apex-anterior deformities in 13% and 19% of cases.[55] Injury to the radial nerve at the time of humeral shaft fracture occurs in approximately 8% to 18% of patients with closed injury.[56] This injury is most common in spiral and transverse fracture patterns.[57] Full recovery of the radial nerve can be expected to occur in 70% of patients treated conservatively over 4 months and approaching 90% overall.[57]

Despite the overall success of conservative management, operative stabilization is necessary in certain fracture and patient types. Gustilo type III injuries, often with gross instability and soft tissue stripping, require irrigation, débridement, and immediate stabilization through internal or external fixation.[55] Patients with ipsilateral brachial plexopathies have been shown to develop nonunion in 45% of a case series of 21 patients.[58] Fracture patterns with proximal extension may fail functional treatment up to 46% of the time and should be observed closely for potential early surgical intervention.[59] Patients who are obese also may have soft tissues that tend to force their alignment into an unacceptable varus deformity and may require early operative intervention.[55]

Surgical Techniques

Intramedullary nail

IMN of diaphyseal humerus fractures has had disappointing outcomes, even with the development of locked nails to control rotation. In theory, the advantage gained from using a load-sharing device with less soft tissue stripping has not borne out improved outcomes. A recent Cochrane review has shown that although functional outcomes are similar between IMN and ORIF methods, hardware removal is significantly more frequent in patients treated with IMN and is most often indicated for shoulder impingement.[60] A randomized prospective study by Putti and colleagues[61] similarly showed that although American Shoulder and Elbow Surgeons scores were similar between IMN and ORIF groups (45.2 and 45.1, respectively), complication rates were significantly higher in the IMN group (50% vs 17%). A meta-analysis comparing plate fixation with IMN demonstrated no difference in infection, nonunion, or radial nerve palsy but a higher incidence of symptomatic shoulder impingement and reoperation was observed with IMN fixation.[62]

Open reduction and internal fixation

ORIF with plate and screw constructs is the mainstay of surgical intervention in humeral shaft fractures when operative intervention is indicated. There has been a substantial focus in the literature on proper fixation techniques for diaphyseal humerus fractures in osteoporotic bone models.

As locked plating technology has been developed, the literature suggests that diaphyseal fracture of the humerus benefit greatly from increased stability of this technology.[63] Initially demonstrated in bone substitute models and redemonstrated in biomechanical studies on matched cadaver constructs, locked or hybrid (mixed locked and unlocked) screw constructs are mechanically superior to unlocked constructs (**Fig. 4**).[63,64] The stiffness of purely locked constructs has been implicated in impaired fracture healing. With hybrid fixation, it is recommended that locked screws be placed on either end of the fracture to attain optimal strength (**Fig. 5**). Furthermore, consideration should be given to the number of screws used in the construct. A recent study has suggested that a 4-screw construct, with 2 cortices above and 2 below the simulated fracture site, had superior resistance to catastrophic failure than a 6-screw construct.[65] In this study it was theorized that the increased screw density created a stress riser, predisposing the 6-screw construct to fail at lighter loads.

Clinical Outcomes and Complications

Successful outcome can be expected after plate fixation of humeral shaft fractures. Even in patients with severely compromised bone quality, union rates after ORIF are reported to be 89%.[66] With the addition of locked plating, patients receiving ORIF after delayed or nonunion healing, rates in 2 case series were 100%.[67,68] Functional scores of patients treated with IMN tend to be lower (13/20 patients with good to excellent results) compared with patients treated with ORIF

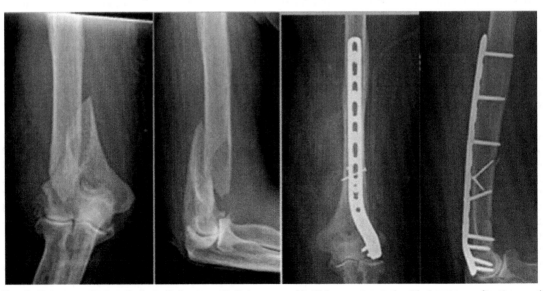

Fig. 4. Osteoporotic humeral shaft fracture (*left two panels*). This was treated with lag screw fixation and a locking neutralization plate (*right two panels*).

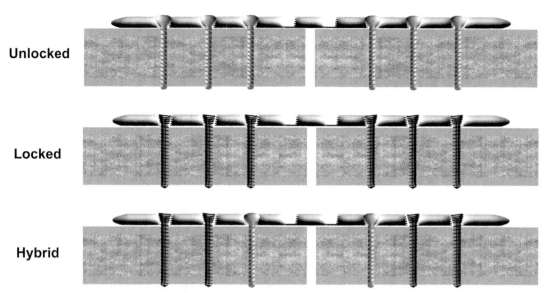

Unlocked

Locked

Hybrid

Fig. 5. Illustration of a hybrid construction using both locked and unlocked screws. (*From* Gardner MJ, Griffith MH, Demetrakopoulos D, et al. Hybrid locked plating of osteoporotic fractures of the humerus. J Bone Joint Surg Am 2006;88:1962–7; with permission.)

(15/16 patients).[69] Injury to the radial nerve is the most devastating complication of humeral shaft fixation. A thorough understanding of anatomy combined with careful retraction, fracture reduction, and plate fixation is required to ensure iatrogenic injury does not occur. The radial nerve crosses the humeral shaft along its' posterior border, approximately 20 cm proximal to the medial epicondyle and 14 cm proximal to the lateral epicondyle, and is frequently encountered during the popular posterior approach.[70] In a series of patients with uninfected nonunions, transient radial nerve palsies were present in 4 of 46 patients postoperatively after revision ORIF. All patients, however, spontaneously recovered radial nerve function.[71]

PROXIMAL FEMUR
Introduction

Fractures of the proximal femur are the most common type of osteoporotic fracture and the one associated with the greatest morbidity and mortality. The majority (>90%) results from a low energy mechanism, such as a fall from a standing height.[72] With the largest generation of Americans now approaching its 7th and 8th decades, the incidence is increasing rapidly. Approximately 280,000 elderly hip fractures occur each year in the United States. Researchers project that by 2040 the annual incidence of hip fractures will approach 500,000.[72] The morbidity and mortality of proximal femur fractures represent a massive burden on the health care system. Mortality in the first year after

hip fracture has been reported as high as 30% and is most often secondary to deep vein thrombosis with pulmonary embolism, pneumonia, and infection.[2] In those patients who survive the perioperative period, only 75% return to prefracture activity level and function. The expense is also significant. Treatment of proximal femur fractures is estimated at $13.8 billion annually.[73]

Fractures of the proximal femur can be divided into 2 major categories: intracapsular and extracapsular. Intracapsular fractures include fractures of the femoral neck and are a common injury in the elderly population. Extracapsular fractures involve the trochanteric and subtrochanteric regions of the femur and extends from the margin of the hip capsule insertion to 5-cm distal to the lesser trochanter on the femoral shaft.[74] The Arbeitsgemeinschaft fur Osteosynthesfragen (AO) classification system separates extracapsular proximal femur fractures into 3 basic types: simple pertrochanteric fractures (31-A1), multifragmentary pertrochanteric fractures (31-A2), and intertrochanteric fractures (31-A3) (**Fig. 6**).[74,75] Fracture classification serves to guide fixation. These fracture types are further classified into stable (A1.1, A1.2, and A2.1) and unstable (A1.3, A2.2, A2.3, and all A3).

Surgical Techniques: Intracapsular Fractures

Screws
Stable intracapsular fractures with nondisplaced or impacted fracture patterns can successfully be treated with percutaneous cannulated screw fixation. The optimal construct involves 3 screws

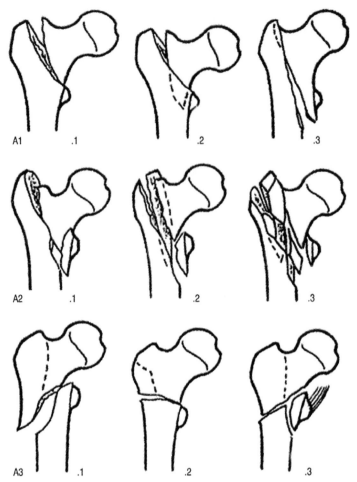

Fig. 6. AO classification of extracapsular proximal femur fractures. (*From* Pervez H, Parker MJ, Pryor GA, et al. Classification of trochanteric fracture of the proximal femur: a study of the reliability of current systems. Injury 2002;33:713–5; with permission.)

placed in an inverted triangle configuration. Positioning of the screw construct inferiorly along the calcar serves to improve fixation strength. The incidence of nonunion varies from 2% to 15%.[76,77]

Arthroplasty

Arthroplasty is a reliable treatment option for elderly patients with displaced intracapsular fractures of the proximal femur. When compared with internal fixation, arthroplasty is associated with improved postoperative function, reduced reoperation rate, and higher patient satisfaction compared with osteosynthesis with internal fixation.[78] Total hip arthroplasty is preferred over hemiarthroplasty in more active older individuals and in those with preexisting arthritis.[79,80] In debilitated patients with significant comorbidities, hemiarthroplasty provides a less invasive option with decreased risk of postoperative dislocation and is preferred over internal fixation.

Surgical Techniques: Extracapsular Fractures

Sliding hip screw

The sliding hip screw is a reliable and inexpensive option for fixation of stable intertrochanteric fractures. The construct is analogous to a lateral tension band, allowing for controlled collapse of the proximal fragment on the medial cortex of the proximal femoral shaft. With fracture collapse, the lever arm is reduced, and forces experienced across the construct are diminished. Critical aspects of surgical technique include the use of a plate between 130° and 150° and a central as well as deep position of the lag screw in the femoral head. As described by Baumgaertner and colleagues,[81] the tip-apex distance (summation of the measurements from the tip of the lag screw to the femoral head in the anteroposterior and lateral views) less than 25 mm correlates with a lower rate of cutout of the lag screw from the femoral head (**Fig. 7**). In addition, De Bruijn

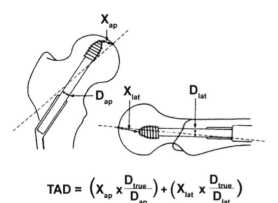

$$TAD = \left(X_{ap} \times \frac{D_{true}}{D_{ap}} \right) + \left(X_{lat} \times \frac{D_{true}}{D_{lat}} \right)$$

Fig. 7. Measurement of tip apex distance. D_{ap}, (Diameter of the lag screw as measured on the anterior-posterior view (mm)); D_{lat}, (True known diameter of the lag screw as measured on the lateral view (mm)); D_{true}, (True known diameter of the lag screw (mm)); TAD, (tip-apex distance); X_{ap}, (Distance from tip of the screw to the apex of the femoral head as measured on anterior-posterior view (mm)); X_{lat}, (Distance from the tip of the screw to the apex of the femoral head as measured on the lateral view (mm)). (*From* Baumgaertner MR, Curtin SL, Lindskog DM, et al. The value of the tip-apex distance in predicting failure of fixation of peritrochanteric fractures of the hip. J Bone Joint Surg Am 1995;77:1058–64; with permission.)

and colleagues[82] suggested that the central-central, anterior-inferior, and central-inferior positions of the screw in the femoral head contribute to protecting the screw from cutout (**Fig. 8**).

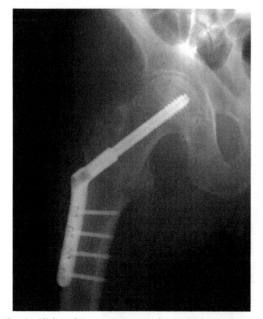

Fig. 8. Sliding hip screw properly position deep and central in the femoral head. (*From* Haidukewych GJ. Intertrochanteric fractures: ten tips to improve results. J Bone Joint Surg Am 2009;91:712–9; with permission.)

Despite reliable fixation in stable fractures, the sliding hip screw has limitations. In the setting of unstable fractures with comminution of the posteromedial proximal femoral cortex, reverse obliquity, or subtrochanteric extension, excessive sliding of the proximal fragment occurs resulting in medialization of the femoral shaft and fixation failure.[83,84]

Cephalomedullary nail

The cephalomedullary nail is another option available for fixation of extracapsular proximal femur fractures. The intramedullary position of the device results in several advantages, including a shortened lever arm, which reduces tensile stress on the implant; a lack of reliance on an intact medial cortex; medial positioning of the implant, which produces more efficient load transfer and shorter operative times; and lower blood loss.[85] The insertion of the IMNs for proximal femur fractures is similar in technique to the standard insertion of a femoral IMN, with fixation secured by a lag screw and distal locking screw. Many clinical trials and biomechanical studies have not shown a significant advantage of the IMN for stable fracture patterns. IMNs are favored, however, in unstable fractures or fractures involving the lateral wall of the greater trochanter.[86,87] Intramedullary fixation of unstable fractures avoids the excessive shortening and medialization of the femoral shaft that can occur after mobilization in patients treated with sliding hip screw constructs. Recent literature also highlights the importance of an intact lateral femoral wall in fracture stability (**Fig. 9**). Intertrochanteric fractures with preoperative or intraoperative fracture of the lateral femoral wall should be treated with IMN because fixation failure and reoperation rates are reduced in comparison to fixation with a sliding hip screw.[83,86] A final advantage of cephalomedullary nail is the shorter operative time and reduced blood loss, which can be beneficial in sick patients with multiple medical comorbidities (**Fig. 10**).

External fixation

As in all traumatic and unstable fracture patterns, external fixation is a possible surgical method to treat osteoporotic proximal femur fractures. External fixation was a popular method of treatment several decades ago but was largely abandoned after the development of improved internal fixation techniques. In addition, external fixation was traditionally associated with complications, such as pin loosening, pin track infections, and varus angulation of the fracture fragments. Recently, however, the development of hydroxyapatite-coated pins has led to a renewed interest in the use of external fixation. In a review by Moroni and colleagues,[73]

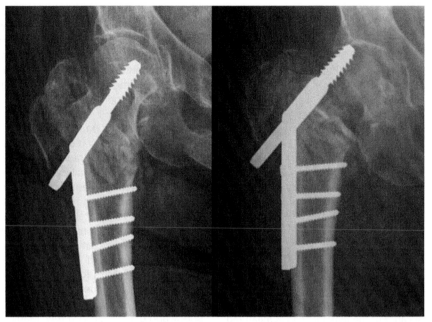

Fig. 9. Fixation failure of sliding hip screw fixation of intertrochanteric fracture with deficient lateral wall. Radiograph immediately following initial fixation (*left*). Follow-up radiograph depicting fixation failure (*right*). (*From* Palm H, Jacobsen S, Sonne-Holm S, et al. Integrity of the lateral femoral wall in intertrochanteric hip fractures: an important predictor of a reoperation. J Bone Joint Surg Am 2007;89:470–5; with permission.)

new generations of external fixation devices have been shown to result in low complication rates and good fixation in osteoporotic bone. This technique has failed to gain widespread popularity but remains a viable option in unstable patients and in patients with comorbid medical conditions who benefit from the minimally invasive approach and shortened operative time.

Clinical Outcomes and Complications

When properly applied, the currently available techniques for surgical fixation of osteoporotic proximal femur fractures can lead to good to excellent outcomes in most patients. In considering all fracture types, approximately greater than 60% to 73% of patients are able to return to prefracture levels of function.[88,89] Poorer outcomes typically

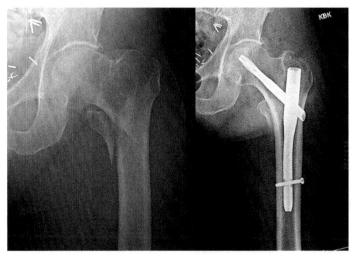

Fig. 10. Unstable intertrochanteric fracture (*left*). This was successfully treated with an intramedullary device.

occur in older patients with multiple comorbidities. Displaced femoral neck fractures treated with arthroplasty result in improved patient outcome and decreased reoperation rates when with internal fixation; however, infection and operative blood loss is increased.[80,90–92] Despite operative treatment, mortality after fracture remains moderate, ranging from 0% to 20% in the first 4 months postoperative months.[90] Nondisplaced intracapsular fracture can be treated with percutaneous screw fixation. Complications of this technique include excessive femoral neck shortening and varus collapse, both of which have been associated with poorer patient-rated outcome.[93,94] Sliding hip screw is the implant of choice for stable intertrochanteric fractures.[95] Failure of the sliding hip screw occurs in approximately 10% cases and is most often secondary to failure to achieve central placement of the screw with excessive tip-apex distance and/or improper implant choice with attempted fixation of unstable fracture types (**Fig. 11**).[81,96] There is no advantage of IMN fixation of stable fractures over the sliding hip screw.[85] First-generation IMNs were associated with increased risk of femur fracture around the implant, but this has been reported less often with second-generation generation.[74] Loss of fixation has occurred with IMNs and, similar to the sliding hip screw, can lead to a varus deformity at the fracture site. Cephalomedullary nailing, however, provides reliable fixation of unstable intertrochanteric

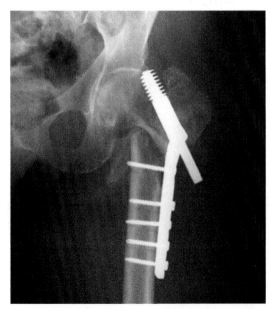

Fig. 11. Failed sliding hip screw fixation of reverse obliquity fracture. (*From* Haidukewych GJ. Intertrochanteric fractures: ten tips to improve results. J Bone Joint Surg Am 2009;91:712–9; with permission.)

fractures of those with reverse obliquity and of those with subtrochanteric extension.

DISTAL FEMUR
Introduction

The distal femur is another common site of osteoporotic fracture. In general, patients who sustain osteoporotic fractures have a higher prevalence of comorbidities, further complicating their care, and an increased postoperative mortality.[97] Reported mortality rates after operative fixation of distal femur fractures range from 2% to 10% at 1 month, 13% to 17% at 6 months, and 23% to 30% at 1 year.[97] These numbers underline the serious implications associated with osteoporotic distal femur fractures.

Treatment of distal femur fractures is almost exclusively operative with nonoperative treatment, resulting in an unacceptably high percentage of patients with nonunion, deformity, and joint stiffness.[98] As with other osteoporotic fractures, the weak, porous metaphyseal bone of the distal femur makes implant fixation a challenge. Several different surgical techniques have been described. Fixation using a blade plate was once the gold standard.[98] The development of locked plate technology and advancements in intramedullary fixation, however, have increased the options available for distal femur fixation.

Surgical Techniques

Blade plate
The fixed-angle blade plate was traditionally the gold standard for distal femur fixation, replacing the extramedullary nonlocked plate. The implant allows for stable fixation in weak osteoporotic bone; however, its application is technically challenging. Given the technical difficulty and the availability of locking plates, blade plates are currently typically used for revision or nonunion situations.

Locked plate fixation
The locking plate was groundbreaking as a fixation device for distal femur fractures in that it offered preservation of soft tissues through a minimally invasive insertion technique and facilitated bridge plating with indirect reduction of comminuted metaphyseal segments.[99] This bridge plating does not obtain interfragmentary compression, and comminuted metaphyseal segments heal through callus formation.[99] The design of the locking plates includes threading in the holes, which allows for locking of the screws, producing a fixed-angle device with angular stability and superior torsional stiffness over other surgical

techniques.[98,100] Biomechanical studies have shown both greater torsional and axial strength for the locking plate over other fixed-angle extramedullary devices, such as the blade plate and the dynamic condylar screw.[98] The torsional strength of the locking plate has made it the most popular extramedullary method of operative fixation for osteoporotic distal femur fractures.

Intramedullary nail

The desire for a minimally invasive surgical technique that provides a stable fixation construct led to development of IMNs. This method became popular for the operative treatment of distal femur fractures in the 1990s for its central implant position.[101] For distal femur fractures, a retrograde IMN is most commonly used for improved distal fixation. Antegrade IMNs are often limited to supracondylar metadiaphyseal distal femur fractures. Retrograde IMNs offer similar advantages to the locking plate construct, which include a minimally invasive insertion technique that limits soft tissue stripping, lower intraoperative blood loss than many fixation procedures, and a biomechanical advantage of central implant position.[102] Also, the retrograde IMN spans the zone of comminution, allowing a multifragmentary fracture pattern to heal with an external callus.[102] One disadvantage of retrograde nailing is that the device cannot be used to assist in fracture reduction, as plates can. Biomechanical analysis of the strength of IMNs has shown that these devices have a greater axial strength than the locking plate constructs, allowing earlier postoperative

mobilization and rehabilitation.[98] The use of 4 interlocking distal screws has been shown to enhance stability and fixation strength when compared with nails with a 1-screw or 2-screw pattern of distal interlocking (**Fig. 12**).[98]

Clinical Outcomes and Complications

Modern-day fixation of osteoporotic distal femurs fractures is most commonly achieved with either locked lateral plating or IMNs. Biomechanical studies have consistently shown that locked plating devices have a greater torsional stiffness than IMNs, whereas the nail constructs have a greater axial strength.[98] These results have profound implications on fracture healing and postoperative clinical outcomes.

There has been recent research devoted to quantifying the callus formation promoted by locking plates and IMNss. The data obtained by these studies have consistently shown that more callus formation is observed in patients treated with IMNs. Several theories exist regarding the lower amount of callus formation in the locking plate constructs. One popular and accepted reason proposes that the stiffness of the locking plates suppresses callus formation.[102] Biomechanical analysis has shown that asymmetric callus often forms with the locking plate system, in which more callus is seen on the medially away from the plate, where more motion occurs.[99,102] This suggests that the excessive stiffness leads to callus suppression, having an impact on fracture healing and potentially causing higher rates of nonunion.[103]

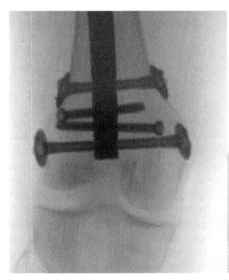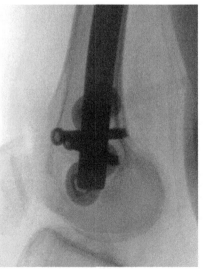

Fig. 12. Distal femur IMN fixation with multiple distal interlocking screws. (*From* Muckley T, Wahnert D, Hoffmeier KL, et al. Internal fixation of type-C distal femoral fractures in osteoporotic bone: surgical technique. J Bone Joint Surg Am 2011;93 Suppl 1:40–53; with permission.)

Herrera and coworkers[104] conducted a systemic review of 415 distal femur fractures and found that locked plating produced a nonunion rate of 5.3% compared with 1.5% from IMNs. Despite the differences in torsional stiffness, axial strength, and callus formation, however, prospective studies have not shown a significant difference in terms of functional outcomes between locked plating and IMNs. Both surgical techniques have the potential to achieve stable fixation and adequate fracture healing, leading to satisfactory clinical outcomes.

SUMMARY

The management of osteoporotic fractures continues to present a challenge to the treating surgeon. As the average age of the populace continues to rise, the burden of fragility fractures is expected to grow as well. It is imperative to recognize the biostructural changes of osteoporotic bone and its implication on fracture fixation. With application of the techniques and implant designs (discussed previously), stable fixation and successful outcome can be achieved in the treatment of many osteoporotic fractures.

REFERENCES

1. Dell RM, Greene D, Anderson D, et al. Osteoporosis disease management: what every orthopaedic surgeon should know. J Bone Joint Surg Am 2009;91(Suppl 6):79–86.
2. Abrahamsen B, van Staa T, Ariely R, et al. Excess mortality following hip fracture: a systematic epidemiological review. Osteoporos Int 2009;20: 1633–50.
3. Willett K, Hearn TC, Cuncins AV. Biomechanical testing of a new design for Schanz pedicle screws. J Orthop Trauma 1993;7:375–80.
4. Turner IG, Rice GN. Comparison of bone screw holding strength in healthy bovine and osteoporotic human cancellous bone. Clin Mater 1992;9: 105–7.
5. Helfet D. Fractures of the distal femur. In: Browner BD, Jupiter JJ, Levine AM, et al, editors. Skeletal trauma: fractures, dislocations, ligamentous injuries. Philadelphia: WB Saunders; 1992. p. 1643–83.
6. Panchbhavi VK, Vallurupalli S, Morris R. Comparison of augmentation methods for internal fixation of osteoporotic ankle fractures. Foot Ankle Int 2009;30:696–703.
7. Moroni A, Toksvig-Larsen S, Maltarello MC, et al. A comparison of hydroxyapatite-coated, titanium-coated, and uncoated tapered external-fixation pins. An in vivo study in sheep. J Bone Joint Surg Am 1998;80:547–54.
8. Agholme F, Andersson T, Tengvall P, et al. Local bisphosphonate release versus hydroxyapatite coating for stainless steel screw fixation in rat tibiae. J Mater Sci Mater Med 2012;23:743–52.
9. Wermelin K, Suska F, Tengvall P, et al. Stainless steel screws coated with bisphosphonates gave stronger fixation and more surrounding bone. Histomorphometry in rats. Bone 2008;42:365–71.
10. Sanders R, Haidukewych GJ, Milne T, et al. Minimal versus maximal plate fixation techniques of the ulna: the biomechanical effect of number of screws and plate length. J Orthop Trauma 2002;16:166–71.
11. Brunner CF, Weber BG. The antiglide plate. In: Brunner CF, Weber BG, editors. Special techniques in internal fixation. New York: Springer-Verlag; 1982. p. 115–33.
12. Egol KA, Kubiak EN, Fulkerson E, et al. Biomechanics of locked plates and screws. J Orthop Trauma 2004;18:488–93.
13. O'Toole RV, Andersen RC, Vesnovsky O, et al. Are locking screws advantageous with plate fixation of humeral shaft fractures? A biomechanical analysis of synthetic and cadaveric bone. J Orthop Trauma 2008;22:709–15.
14. Sommer C, Gautier E, Muller M, et al. First clinical results of the Locking Compression Plate (LCP). Injury 2003;34(Suppl 2):B43–54.
15. Bottlang M, Doornink J, Byrd GD, et al. A nonlocking end screw can decrease fracture risk caused by locked plating in the osteoporotic diaphysis. J Bone Joint Surg Am 2009;91: 620–7.
16. Bottlang M, Doornink J, Lujan TJ, et al. Effects of construct stiffness on healing of fractures stabilized with locking plates. J Bone Joint Surg Am 2010; 92(Suppl 2):12–22.
17. Bottlang M, Doornink J, Fitzpatrick DC, et al. Far cortical locking can reduce stiffness of locked plating constructs while retaining construct strength. J Bone Joint Surg Am 2009;91:1985–94.
18. Doornink J, Fitzpatrick DC, Madey SM, et al. Far cortical locking enables flexible fixation with periarticular locking plates. J Orthop Trauma 2011; 25(Suppl 1):S29–34.
19. Gardner MJ, Nork SE, Huber P, et al. Less rigid stable fracture fixation in osteoporotic bone using locked plates with near cortical slots. Injury 2010; 41:652–6.
20. Gardner MJ, Nork SE, Huber P, et al. Stiffness modulation of locking plate constructs using near cortical slotted holes: a preliminary study. J Orthop Trauma 2009;23:281–7.
21. Sellei RM, Garrison RL, Kobbe P, et al. Effects of near cortical slotted holes in locking plate constructs. J Orthop Trauma 2011;25(Suppl 1): S35–40.

22. Doornink J, Fitzpatrick DC, Boldhaus S, et al. Effects of hybrid plating with locked and nonlocked screws on the strength of locked plating constructs in the osteoporotic diaphysis. J Trauma 2010;69: 411–7.

23. Freeman AL, Tornetta P 3rd, Schmidt A, et al. How much do locked screws add to the fixation of "hybrid" plate constructs in osteoporotic bone? J Orthop Trauma 2010;24:163–9.

24. Kummer FJ, Koval KJ, Kauffman JI. Improving the distal fixation of intramedullary nails in osteoporotic bone. Bull Hosp Jt Dis 1997;56:88–90.

25. Ito K, Hungerbuhler R, Wahl D, et al. Improved intramedullary nail interlocking in osteoporotic bone. J Orthop Trauma 2001;15:192–6.

26. McLaurin TM. Proximal humerus fractures in the elderly are we operating on too many? Bull Hosp Jt Dis 2004;62:24–32.

27. Maravic M, Le Bihan C, Landais P, et al. Incidence and cost of osteoporotic fractures in France during 2001. A methodological approach by the national hospital database. Osteoporos Int 2005; 16:1475–80.

28. Duparc F, Muller JM, Freger P. Arterial blood supply of the proximal humeral epiphysis. Surg Radiol Anat 2001;23:185–90.

29. Neviaser AS, Hettrich CM, Dines JS, et al. Rate of avascular necrosis following proximal humerus fractures treated with a lateral locking plate and endosteal implant. Arch Orthop Trauma Surg 2011;131:1617–22.

30. Crosby LA, Finnan RP, Anderson CG, et al. Tetracycline labeling as a measure of humeral head viability after 3- or 4-part proximal humerus fracture. J Shoulder Elbow Surg 2009;18:851–8.

31. Yang H, Li Z, Zhou F, et al. A prospective clinical study of proximal humerus fractures treated with a locking proximal humerus plate. J Orthop Trauma 2011;25:11–7.

32. Keener JD, Parsons BO, Flatow EL, et al. Outcomes after percutaneous reduction and fixation of proximal humeral fractures. J Shoulder Elbow Surg 2007;16:330–8.

33. Harrison AK, Gruson KI, Zmistowski B, et al. Intermediate outcomes following percutaneous fixation of proximal humeral fractures. J Bone Joint Surg Am 2012;94:1223–8.

34. Jo MJ, Gardner MJ. Proximal humerus fractures. Curr Rev Musculoskelet Med 2012;5(3):192–8.

35. Zhu Y, Lu Y, Shen J, et al. Locking intramedullary nails and locking plates in the treatment of two-part proximal humeral surgical neck fractures: a prospective randomized trial with a minimum of three years of follow-up. J Bone Joint Surg Am 2011;93:159–68.

36. Hatzidakis AM, Shevlin MJ, Fenton DL, et al. Angular-stable locked intramedullary nailing of two-part surgical neck fractures of the proximal part of the humerus. A multicenter retrospective observational study. J Bone Joint Surg Am 2011; 93:2172–9.

37. Ring D. Current concepts in plate and screw fixation of osteoporotic proximal humerus fractures. Injury 2007;38(Suppl 3):S59–68.

38. Gardner MJ, Weil Y, Barker JU, et al. The importance of medial support in locked plating of proximal humerus fractures. J Orthop Trauma 2007; 21:185–91.

39. Egol KA, Sugi MT, Ong CC, et al. Fracture site augmentation with calcium phosphate cement reduces screw penetration after open reduction-internal fixation of proximal humeral fractures. J Shoulder Elbow Surg 2012;21:741–8.

40. Gardner MJ, Boraiah S, Helfet DL, et al. Indirect medial reduction and strut support of proximal humerus fractures using an endosteal implant. J Orthop Trauma 2008;22:195–200.

41. Neviaser AS, Hettrich CM, Beamer BS, et al. Endosteal strut augment reduces complications associated with proximal humeral locking plates. Clin Orthop Relat Res 2011;469:3300–6.

42. Neer CS 2nd. Displaced proximal humeral fractures. II. Treatment of three-part and four-part displacement. J Bone Joint Surg Am 1970;52: 1090–103.

43. Boileau P, Krishnan SG, Tinsi L, et al. Tuberosity malposition and migration: reasons for poor outcomes after hemiarthroplasty for displaced fractures of the proximal humerus. J Shoulder Elbow Surg 2002;11:401–12.

44. Inauen C, Platz A, Meier C, et al. Quality of Life after Osteosynthesis of Fractures of the Proximal Humerus. J Orthop Trauma 2012. [Epub ahead of print].

45. Solberg BD, Moon CN, Franco DP, et al. Surgical treatment of three and four-part proximal humeral fractures. J Bone Joint Surg Am 2009;91:1689–97.

46. Owsley KC, Gorczyca JT. Fracture displacement and screw cutout after open reduction and locked plate fixation of proximal humeral fractures [corrected]. J Bone Joint Surg Am 2008;90:233–40.

47. Paolieri D, Lotto L, Leoncini D, et al. Differential effects of grammatical gender and gender inflection in bare noun production. Br J Psychol 2011; 102:19–36.

48. Murray IR, Amin AK, White TO, et al. Proximal humeral fractures: current concepts in classification, treatment and outcomes. J Bone Joint Surg Br 2011;93:1–11.

49. Konrad G, Bayer J, Hepp P, et al. Open reduction and internal fixation of proximal humeral fractures with use of the locking proximal humerus plate. Surgical technique. J Bone Joint Surg Am 2010; 92(Suppl 1 Pt 1):85–95.

50. Sudkamp N, Bayer J, Hepp P, et al. Open reduction and internal fixation of proximal humeral fractures with use of the locking proximal humerus plate. Results of a prospective, multicenter, observational study. J Bone Joint Surg Am 2009;91: 1320–8.

51. Zhu Y, Lu Y, Wang M, et al. Treatment of proximal humeral fracture with a proximal humeral nail. J Shoulder Elbow Surg 2010;19:297–302.

52. Robinson CM, Page RS, Hill RM, et al. Primary hemiarthroplasty for treatment of proximal humeral fractures. J Bone Joint Surg Am 2003;85-A:1215–23.

53. Ekholm R, Adami J, Tidermark J, et al. Fractures of the shaft of the humerus. An epidemiological study of 401 fractures. J Bone Joint Surg Br 2006;88: 1469–73.

54. Tytherleigh-Strong G, Walls N, McQueen MM. The epidemiology of humeral shaft fractures. J Bone Joint Surg Br 1998;80:249–53.

55. Sarmiento A, Zagorski JB, Zych GA, et al. Functional bracing for the treatment of fractures of the humeral diaphysis. J Bone Joint Surg Am 2000; 82:478–86.

56. Pollock FH, Drake D, Bovill EG, et al. Treatment of radial neuropathy associated with fractures of the humerus. J Bone Joint Surg Am 1981;63:239–43.

57. Shao YC, Harwood P, Grotz MR, et al. Radial nerve palsy associated with fractures of the shaft of the humerus: a systematic review. J Bone Joint Surg Br 2005;87:1647–52.

58. Brien WW, Gellman H, Becker V, et al. Management of fractures of the humerus in patients who have an injury of the ipsilateral brachial plexus. J Bone Joint Surg Am 1990;72:1208–10.

59. Toivanen JA, Nieminen J, Laine HJ, et al. Functional treatment of closed humeral shaft fractures. Int Orthop 2005;29:10–3.

60. Kurup H, Hossain M, Andrew JG. Dynamic compression plating versus locked intramedullary nailing for humeral shaft fractures in adults. Cochrane Database Syst Rev 2011;(6):CD005959.

61. Putti AB, Uppin RB, Putti BB. Locked intramedullary nailing versus dynamic compression plating for humeral shaft fractures. J Orthop Surg 2009; 17(2):139–41.

62. Bhandari M, Devereaux PJ, McKee MD, et al. Compression plating versus intramedullary nailing of humeral shaft fractures–a meta-analysis. Acta Orthop 2006;77:279–84.

63. Davis C, Stall A, Knutsen E, et al. Locking plates in osteoporosis: a biomechanical cadaveric study of diaphyseal humerus fractures. J Orthop Trauma 2012;26:216–21.

64. Gardner MJ, Griffith MH, Demetrakopoulos D, et al. Hybrid locked plating of osteoporotic fractures of the humerus. J Bone Joint Surg Am 2006;88: 1962–7.

65. Hak DJ, Althausen P, Hazelwood SJ. Locked plate fixation of osteoporotic humeral shaft fractures: are two locking screws per segment enough? J Orthop Trauma 2010;24:207–11.

66. Wright TW. Treatment of humeral diaphyseal nonunions in patients with severely compromised bone. J South Orthop Assoc 1997;6:1–7.

67. Wenzl ME, Porte T, Fuchs S, et al. Delayed and non-union of the humeral diaphysis—compression plate or internal plate fixator? Injury 2004; 35:55–60.

68. Ring D, Kloen P, Kadzielski J, et al. Locking compression plates for osteoporotic nonunions of the diaphyseal humerus. Clin Orthop Relat Res 2004;(425):50–4.

69. Singisetti K, Ambedkar M. Nailing versus plating in humerus shaft fractures: a prospective comparative study. Int Orthop 2010;34:571–6.

70. Gerwin M, Hotchkiss RN, Weiland AJ. Alternative operative exposures of the posterior aspect of the humeral diaphysis with reference to the radial nerve. J Bone Joint Surg Am 1996;78:1690–5.

71. Abalo A, Dosseh ED, Adabra K, et al. Open reduction and internal fixation of humeral non-unions: radiological and functional results. Acta Orthop Belg 2011;77:299–303.

72. National Hospital Discharge Survey (NHDS). In: Statistics TNCfH, edition. 2010.

73. Moroni A, Faldini C, Pegreffi F, et al. Osteoporotic pertrochanteric fractures can be successfully treated with external fixation. J Bone Joint Surg Am 2005;87(Suppl 2):42–51.

74. Parker MJ, Handoll HH. Gamma and other cephalocondylic intramedullary nails versus extramedullary implants for extracapsular hip fractures in adults. Cochrane Database Syst Rev 2005;19(14): CD000093.

75. Pervez H, Parker MJ, Pryor GA, et al. Classification of trochanteric fracture of the proximal femur: a study of the reliability of current systems. Injury 2002;33:713–5.

76. Bray TJ, Chapman MW. Percutaneous pinning of intracapsular hip fractures. Instr Course Lect 1984;33:168–79.

77. Chiu KY, Pun WK, Luk KD, et al. Cancellous screw fixation for subcapital femoral neck fractures. J R Coll Surg Edinb 1994;39:130–2.

78. Gjertsen JE, Vinje T, Engesaeter LB, et al. Internal screw fixation compared with bipolar hemiarthroplasty for treatment of displaced femoral neck fractures in elderly patients. J Bone Joint Surg Am 2010;92:619–28.

79. Blomfeldt R, Tornkvist H, Ponzer S, et al. Comparison of internal fixation with total hip replacement for displaced femoral neck fractures. Randomized, controlled trial performed at four years. J Bone Joint Surg Am 2005;87:1680–8.

80. Healy WL, Iorio R. Total hip arthroplasty: optimal treatment for displaced femoral neck fractures in elderly patients. Clin Orthop Relat Res 2004;(429):43–8.

81. Baumgaertner MR, Curtin SL, Lindskog DM, et al. The value of the tip-apex distance in predicting failure of fixation of peritrochanteric fractures of the hip. J Bone Joint Surg Am 1995;77:1058–64.

82. De Bruijn K, den Hartog D, Tuinebreijer W, et al. Reliability of predictors for screw cutout in intertrochanteric hip fractures. J Bone Joint Surg Am 2012;94:1266–72.

83. Haidukewych GJ. Intertrochanteric fractures: ten tips to improve results. J Bone Joint Surg Am 2009;91:712–9.

84. Lorich DG, Geller DS, Nielson JH. Osteoporotic pertrochanteric hip fractures: management and current controversies. Instr Course Lect 2004;53: 441–54.

85. Saudan M, Lubbeke A, Sadowski C, et al. Pertrochanteric fractures: is there an advantage to an intramedullary nail? A randomized, prospective study of 206 patients comparing the dynamic hip screw and proximal femoral nail. J Orthop Trauma 2002;16:386–93.

86. Palm H, Jacobsen S, Sonne-Holm S, et al. Integrity of the lateral femoral wall in intertrochanteric hip fractures: an important predictor of a reoperation. J Bone Joint Surg Am 2007;89:470–5.

87. Palm H, Krasheninnikoff M, Holck K, et al. A new algorithm for hip fracture surgery. Reoperation rate reduced from 18 % to 12 % in 2,000 consecutive patients followed for 1 year. Acta Orthop 2003; 83:26–30.

88. Iorio R, Healy WL, Appleby D, et al. Displaced femoral neck fractures in the elderly: disposition and outcome after 3- to 6-year follow-up evaluation. J Arthroplasty 2004;19:175–9.

89. Koval KJ, Skovron ML, Aharonoff GB, et al. Predictors of functional recovery after hip fracture in the elderly. Clin Orthop Relat Res 1998;(348):22–8.

90. Bhandari M, Devereaux PJ, Swiontkowski MF, et al. Internal fixation compared with arthroplasty for displaced fractures of the femoral neck. A meta-analysis. J Bone Joint Surg Am 2003;85-A: 1673–81.

91. Gao H, Liu Z, Xing D, et al. Which is the best alternative for displaced femoral neck fractures in the elderly? A meta-analysis. Clin Orthop Relat Res 2012;470:1782–91.

92. Rogmark C, Johnell O. Primary arthroplasty is better than internal fixation of displaced femoral neck fractures: a meta-analysis of 14 randomized studies with 2,289 patients. Acta Orthop 2006;77: 359–67.

93. Zlowodzki M, Brink O, Switzer J, et al. The effect of shortening and varus collapse of the femoral neck on function after fixation of intracapsular fracture of the hip: a multi-centre cohort study. J Bone Joint Surg Br 2008;90:1487–94.

94. Weil YA, Khoury A, Zuaiter I, et al. Femoral neck shortening and varus collapse after navigated fixation of intracapsular femoral neck fractures. J Orthop Trauma 2012;26:19–23.

95. Parker MJ, Handoll HH. Gamma and other cephalocondylic intramedullary nails versus extramedullary implants for extracapsular hip fractures in adults. Cochrane Database Syst Rev 2008;(3): CD000093.

96. Audige L, Hanson B, Swiontkowski MF. Implant-related complications in the treatment of unstable intertrochanteric fractures: meta-analysis of dynamic screw-plate versus dynamic screw-intramedullary nail devices. Int Orthop 2003;27: 197–203.

97. Streubel PN, Ricci WM, Wong A, et al. Mortality after distal femur fractures in elderly patients. Clin Orthop Relat Res 2011;469:1188–96.

98. Muckley T, Wahnert D, Hoffmeier KL, et al. Internal fixation of type-C distal femoral fractures in osteoporotic bone: surgical technique. J Bone Joint Surg Am 2011;93(Suppl 1):40–53.

99. Lujan TJ, Henderson CE, Madey SM, et al. Locked plating of distal femur fractures leads to inconsistent and asymmetric callus formation. J Orthop Trauma 2010;24:156–62.

100. Cornell CN, Ayalon O. Evidence for success with locking plates for fragility fractures. HSS J 2011; 7:164–9.

101. Henderson CE, Kuhl LL, Fitzpatrick DC, et al. Locking plates for distal femur fractures: is there a problem with fracture healing? J Orthop Trauma 2011;25(Suppl 1):S8–14.

102. Henderson CE, Lujan T, Bottlang M, et al. Stabilization of distal femur fractures with intramedullary nails and locking plates: differences in callus formation. Iowa Orthop J 2010;30:61–8.

103. Henderson CE, Lujan TJ, Kuhl LL, et al. 2010 mid-America Orthopaedic Association Physician in Training Award: healing complications are common after locked plating for distal femur fractures. Clin Orthop Relat Res 2011;469:1757–65.

104. Herrera DA, Kregor PJ, Cole PA, et al. Treatment of acute distal femur fractures above a total knee arthroplasty: systematic review of 415 cases (1981-2006). Acta Orthop 2008;79:22–7.

The Osteoporotic Acetabular Fracture

Patrick D.G. Henry, MD, FRCSC[a],[*],
Hans J. Kreder, MD, MPH, FRCSC[b],
Richard J. Jenkinson, MD, MSc, FRCSC[a]

KEYWORDS

- Geriatric acetabular fracture • Fragility fracture • Arthroplasty • Osteoporosis

KEY POINTS

- Twenty-four percent of acetabular fractures occur in patients older than 60 years, and this proportion is increasing.
- Prolonged traction or bed rest is never indicated for these injuries, especially in the medically ill patient.
- Treatment options include:
  - Nonoperative management with early mobilization
  - Open reduction and internal fixation with standard or minimally invasive techniques
  - With or without planned delayed total hip arthroplasty
  - Acute total hip arthroplasty in selected patients
- Treatment choices need to be individualized based on fracture characteristics, patients' physiologic age, and functional demands.

INTRODUCTION

Emile Letournel's original text on acetabular fractures was published in 1964. He listed one of the contraindications to acetabular fracture surgery as age older than 60 years.[1] However, in the second edition, age was removed as a contraindication to surgery. Changes to Letournel's text reflect a shift in orthopedic evaluation and treatment of the elderly. Geriatric patients 65 years and older are the fastest growing demographic of acetabular fractures.[2] These individuals are becoming increasingly active, better informed, and often have high expectations for their health outcomes.[3] Prolonged bed rest, especially with the addition of traction, is particularly harmful to elderly patients.[4] All elderly patients with acetabular fracture need a treatment plan that involves early mobilization, and for the vast majority of independent patients with displaced fractures, surgical management is recommended.[5,6]

The bulk of literature on osteoporosis has focused on fractures of the proximal femur vertebra, humerus, and wrist.[7–14] Acknowledgment of acetabular fractures as true fragility fractures has been slow, and the provision of appropriate solutions even slower.[15] A recent systematic review identified a major gap between basic science research on bone quality and translation to evidence-based clinical practice.[16] This observation is particularly applicable to fragility fractures of the acetabulum, for which there is a paucity of literature.

Funding Sources: Nil (P.D.G.H., R.J.J.); Departmental research support from Biomet, Zimmer (H.J.K.).
Conflict of Interest: None.
^a Division of Orthopaedics, Department of Surgery, Sunnybrook Health Science Center, University of Toronto, Room MG 314, 2075 Bayview Avenue, Toronto, Ontario M4N 3M5, Canada; ^b Orthopaedic Surgery and Health Policy Evaluation & Management, Division of Orthopaedic Surgery, Sunnybrook Health Science Centre, University of Toronto, Room MG 314, 2075 Bayview Avenue, Toronto, Ontario M4N 3M5, Canada
* Corresponding author.
E-mail address: drpdghenry@gmail.com

Orthop Clin N Am 44 (2013) 201–215
http://dx.doi.org/10.1016/j.ocl.2013.01.002
0030-5898/13/$ – see front matter © 2013 Elsevier Inc. All rights reserved.

orthopedic.theclinics.com

THE PROBLEM: AN EXPANDING ELDERLY POPULATION, OSTEOPOROSIS, AND LOW-ENERGY ACETABULAR FRACTURES

In 1998 the World Health Organization described a "fragility fracture" as a fracture caused by injury that would be insufficient to fracture a normal bone.[17] Since that time, despite an expanding body of literature and education on the subject of osteoporosis, the expanding elderly population has led to a dramatic increase in these injuries.

With an annual incidence of approximately 240,000 per year in the United States,[2] fractures of the proximal femur (hip fractures) are widely regarded as the most devastating of all fragility fractures, with an overall 1-year mortality between 8.4% and 36%.[18] Low-energy acetabular fractures occur less frequently (about 4000 per year in the United States)[2]; however, they have been associated with a similar 1-year mortality of up to 13.9%.[19,20] The rate of surgical fixation of acetabular fractures in the elderly is also increasing. A recent epidemiologic study involving 1309 patients at a Level I trauma center reported the mean age of patients with surgically treated acetabular fractures to have increased from 32 to 49 years, with the proportion of patients older than 60 more than doubled (from 10% to 24%).[21]

FRACTURE MORPHOLOGY

Geriatric acetabular fractures can be either low-energy or high-energy injuries. In elderly patients, between 50% and 83% of acetabular fractures are caused by a simple fall from a standing height onto the affected side, a mechanism shared by most elderly fractures of the proximal femur.[21,22] Rather than fracturing at the femoral neck or intertrochanteric region, these low-energy acetabular fractures occur in a typical pattern (**Fig. 1**):

- Impact of the greater trochanter onto the ground generates an anteromedial force transmission, driving the femoral head into the acetabular socket.[23]
- Anterior column displacement occurs in 64% of cases, compared with only 43% in younger patients with acetabular fractures.[21]
- Using Letournel's classification system, the most common pattern is the anterior

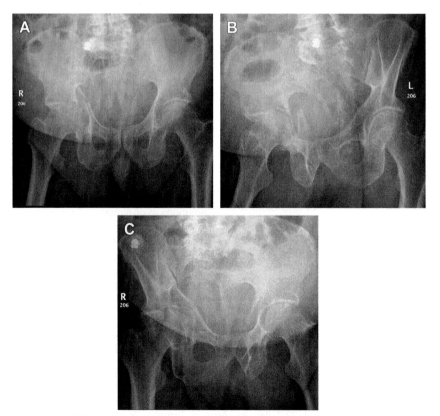

Fig. 1. (*A*) Note the typical features of the geriatric acetabular fracture, including involvement of the anterior column and quadrilateral plate, medial displacement of the femoral head, roof impaction (gull sign), and femoral head injury. (*B*) Iliac oblique view shows better definition of quadrilateral plate displacement. (*C*) Obturator oblique view accentuates anterior column displacement and medialized femoral head.

column/anterior wall, with the second most common being the anterior column posterior hemitransverse pattern with medial protrusion of the femoral head.[21,24–26]

In terms of fracture complexity, the classification system may be somewhat misleading in these patients. As is typical of all osteoporotic fractures, fragile cortices and weakened trabecular bone give way to cortical comminution and metaphyseal impaction, particularly with increasing energy of the injury.[16,27] This process results in 2 of the most commonly reported features of geriatric acetabular fractures: marginal impaction and quadrilateral plate displacement.

- Marginal impaction. This feature is present in approximately 40% of all fractures types, and can involve the radiologic roof (anteromedial or posteromedial articular surfaces).[21] The double density observed on plain radiographs represents impaction of the anteromedial articular surface and has been referred to as the "gull sign" by some investigators (see **Fig. 1**A)[19]; however, careful radiologic and computed tomographic evaluation demonstrates that it is more commonly the posteromedial acetabular surface that experiences impaction, even with anterior column displacement.[21] Moreover, a double density may simply represent overlap of a displaced, nonimpacted, anterior fragment superimposed on the intact dome.
- Quadrilateral plate displacement. In the series of 235 patients older than 60 years with operatively treated acetabular fractures evaluated by Ferguson and colleagues,[21] displacement and comminution of the quadrilateral plate was present in more than half of cases, and was more common with anterior column displacement. Once the thin cortical bone of the quadrilateral plate is disrupted,

with continued force, the femoral head follows the displaced anterior column and comes to rest medial to the native acetabulum, creating so-called intrapelvic dislocation (**Fig. 2**A),[23,27,28] frequently damaging the femoral-head cartilage during this process (see **Fig. 1**A).[2,19,21,29]

TREATMENT

There are two important goals when managing any fragility fracture: Appropriate care for the acute fracture, and prevention of secondary fractures. Whereas orthopedic surgeons have traditionally focused on the former, initiatives such as the American Academy of Orthopaedic Surgeons "Own the Bone" program have demonstrated that by taking ownership of the latter, orthopedic surgeons can much more dramatically improve long-term health outcomes in these patients.[9,30–33]

Management of Acute Fracture

Goals of treatment are conceptualized into 3 tenets:

- Early mobilization and pain control to prevent complications of bed rest and recumbency
- Optimization of hip-joint function
- Minimize complications from surgical or nonsurgical treatment

Before deliberating the various surgical options, the first priority is to decide whether an operation is warranted. Several considerations are at play in making this decision.

- Several investigators have cautioned against nonoperative management of elderly acetabular fractures,[34–36] having observed poor radiologic, clinical and functional outcomes in 25% to 33% of their nonoperative elderly acetabular fracture patients, with early

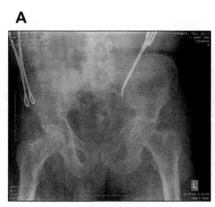
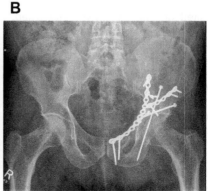

Fig. 2. (A) Intrapelvic dislocation. (B) Anterior column/quadrilateral plate buttress plate.

development of hip-joint arthritis.[35,36] However, the decision process for determining operative versus nonoperative treatment was not detailed.

- As elderly patients have demonstrated a clinical resilience in the face of poor radiographic outcomes in other anatomic areas such as the distal radius,[37] proximal humerus,[38,39] and supracondylar femur,[40] it is possible that this would be the case with acetabular fractures as well. However, evidence suggests that for acetabular fractures poor anatomic restoration is associated with poor clinical and functional outcome.[21,41]
- Many geriatric patients have limited preinjury mobility, and often have multiple medical comorbidities. The surgical insult of reconstructive acetabular surgery is often significant, may be poorly tolerated by geriatric patients, and may unnecessarily further jeopardize patients' overall health status.

Acetabular fractures in the elderly are commonly unstable injuries that feature involvement of the weight-bearing dome, quadrilateral plate with intrapelvic dislocation, or comminuted posterior wall fractures with posterior instability.[22,23,29,42,43] These types of fractures will not do well under nonoperative management for 2 main reasons:

1. Attempts at mobilization will cause pain and further displacement, making avoidance of bed rest impossible. Complications of bed rest in this age group are well documented.[4,44]
2. Wide displacement and motion at the fracture site will likely lead to severe malunion or nonunion, which will impair later hip function and greatly complicate future salvage arthroplasty.

Nonoperative management is considered for patients with:

- Minimally displaced and/or stable fractures
- Concentric hip joint
- Very limited preinjury functional status (eg, nonambulatory)
- Severe medical comorbidities; patients who are or unlikely to tolerate a surgical procedure

If nonoperative treatment is chosen, the patient should be mobilized to avoid the complications associated with prolonged bed rest. If the patient is able to comply, protected weight bearing may be possible. However, demented or uncooperative patients can only be mobilized "bed to chair." The patient in **Fig. 9**A was treated nonoperatively because of inability to mobilize with partial weight-bearing restrictions and unwillingness to consent to surgery owing to the risk of comorbidities.

A consideration for geriatric acetabular fractures treated nonoperatively is the option of a delayed, usually satisfactory, salvage total hip arthroplasty (THA). Acute THA can be a challenging procedure, as expertise in both acetabular fracture fixation and revision hip arthroplasty is required. Planned staged hip arthroplasty after nonoperative or limited operative treatment is another strategy that may be used. The choice between nonoperative, delayed THA, or acute THA needs to be individualized based on the patient and the expertise available by the treating orthopedic team. A patient with a completely incongruous hip joint should be considered for immediate fracture fixation and concomitant total hip replacement so that the patient can be mobilized as soon as possible (these patients can usually be capable of weight bearing as tolerated). In a more congruous hip joint with which the patient is able to mobilize without excessive pain, delayed total hip replacement can be considered after the fracture has healed to some degree (ideally 12 weeks or more). The only real benefit of delayed total hip replacement is that fracture fixation is not as critical (because of some fracture healing), so that the surgery is less extensive than when the total hip replacement is done acutely.

Standard Open Reduction and Internal Fixation

The aim of open reduction and internal fixation (ORIF) for acetabular fractures is to achieve anatomic restoration of the native joint surface and maintain concentric reduction of the hip joint. These surgical goals are designed to help reduce the risk of postoperative pain, arthritis, and implant failure while maximizing return of function and avoiding subsequent procedures. As with displaced fractures in younger patients, standard approaches (Kocher-Langenbeck, ilioinguinal, or anterior intrapelvic approach [Stoppa]), are selected based on fracture personality. In the majority of cases, a single exposure can be used. Extensile exposures such as the extended iliofemoral approach are best avoided in the elderly, but occasionally combined anterior and posterior approaches (sequential or simultaneous) are required to address articular comminution that cannot be addressed by the main exposure. Each patient's radiographs are critically reviewed, and the surgical approach selected to provide the best exposure for achieving accurate reductions, clamp placement, and fixation.

Once exposure is achieved and a reduction obtained, achieving adequate fixation in the face of osteoporotic bone is a major challenge.[44–47] If the comminuted fragments can be reduced accurately and stable fixation applied, the race against fixation failure has begun. Unfortunately, the altered biological environment of osteoporotic bone has an impaired capacity for robust healing.[44,46] Certain surgical techniques to manage some of these challenges have been described.

- Lag screws alone are inadequate in osteoporotic bone; neutralization plates for column fixation are required.[45] In all cases, buttress plates are required for wall-fracture fixation.
- Although locking implants have advantages in osteoporotic bone, the unusual geometry of the pelvis and acetabulum as well as the need to direct screws at various acute angles limits the use of locking implants in acetabular surgery.[24]
- In a biomechanics article, Culemann and colleagues[24] demonstrated that reinforcement of the quadrilateral plate to prevent persistent femoral-head protrusion was best achieved with standard reconstruction plates, with no advantage imparted by either an "h-plate" or locking plates (the latter due to inability to angle the screws appropriately).
- The Stoppa approach was shown to be particularly advantageous in cases involving the typical medial quadrilateral plate displacement, as it provides superior access to

the quadrilateral plate and also permits placement of intrapelvic plates to buttress this area (**Fig. 3**).[43,47]

The use of standard techniques and wide exposures may be particularly helpful when attempting anatomic reductions in the face of the common morphologic complexities of geriatric fractures, as already described. However, the increased morbidity of wide exposures in medically compromised patients should be balanced with reduction goals, particularly when working with comminuted, osteoporotic bone for which anatomic reduction and fixation may not be possible. In some cases, an imperfect articular reduction may be acceptable if the columns are reduced sufficiently to promote healing, and thus render early mobilization and subsequent THA more technically feasible. Working on this premise, minimally invasive surgical approaches (MIS) become an attractive option.

Minimally Invasive Open Reduction and Internal Fixation

Minimally invasive techniques for fracture fixation have the advantage of reducing the surgical insult to the patient but the disadvantage of providing limited anatomic access to achieve reductions and apply hardware (**Fig. 4**). Thus an anatomic reduction is rarely possible.

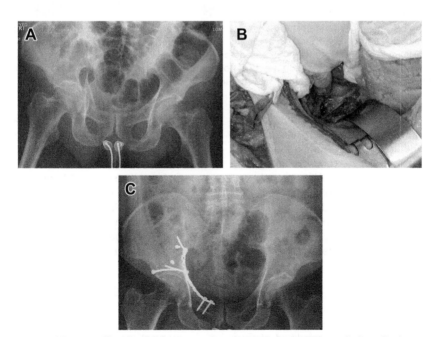

Fig. 3. (*A*) A 68-year-old man suffered a fall from standing, leading to quadrilateral plate displacement. (*B*) Intraoperative photograph demonstrating visualization of quadrilateral plate through anterior intrapelvic approach (Stoppa). (*C*) Buttress plate applied to quadrilateral plate.

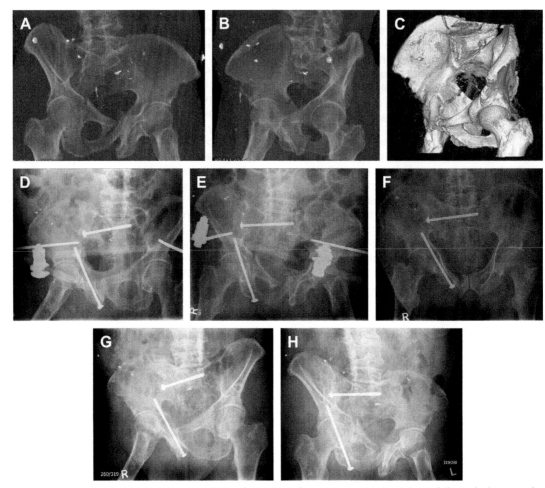

Fig. 4. (*A–C*) Typical T-type geriatric acetabular fracture with anterior column and quadrilateral plate involvement in a 67-year-old man who suffered an acute myocardial infarction at the time of injury. A pelvic fracture is also present. Percutaneous strategies were used to achieve fixation. (*D–F*) Immediate postoperative films. Acetabular reduction was deemed adequate, but nonanatomic. (*G, H*) Four years postoperatively at latest follow-up. The patient was fully ambulatory with minimal hip discomfort.

- Jeffcoat and colleagues[26] evaluated the anterior ilioinguinal (AII) for exposing geriatric acetabular fractures, and demonstrated shorter surgical times and less blood loss using only 2 of the 3 windows of the AII approach, but equivalent functional outcomes as measured by the Short-Form 36 and Musculoskeletal Functional Assessment scores. In this series, the quality of reduction was gauged as similar between the 2 groups, despite the smaller incisions.
- Starr and colleagues[48] have acknowledged a diminished capacity to achieve anatomic reductions, but favorable outcomes with MIS techniques involving stab incisions, the use of ball-spike pushers, and modified clamps to achieve reductions, followed by percutaneous screw fixation. In the cases selected for this treatment, surgical goals were oriented toward limiting soft-tissue dissection while still achieving fracture stabilization, at the sacrifice of anatomic reduction.
- Outcomes using MIS techniques have been comparable with reported outcomes using standard ORIF techniques on geriatric acetabular fractures, although patient selection has been noted to play a critical role in the decision to use MIS techniques.[20,48,49]

There are several attractive elements to an MIS approach, although special expertise and equipment is required:

- Such techniques (presumably) inflict a smaller surgical insult to an already compromised elderly patient with low physiologic reserve, thus lowering the risk of cardiovascular complications caused by the surgery and increasing the chances that the patient will be able to get out of bed and mobilize earlier.

- The geriatric population may tolerate a poor reduction better than the younger population.[5,49]
  - Even in the most experienced hands, anatomic reductions of displaced acetabular fractures are rarely achievable with percutaneous techniques.[48]
  - However, if stability can be achieved percutaneously, then it may be true that articular incongruity is relatively well tolerated by this population.
  - The potential reasons for this are multifactorial, such as a lower functional demand, higher pain tolerance, lower expectations, and a slower progression of arthritis and joint pain.
- If a nonanatomic reduction contributes to rapid arthritic deterioration, arthroplasty is highly successful in this age group, whereas in younger patients prosthetic wear and early failure are a common problem; thus the prevention of arthritis in the younger age group is more crucial.[50,51]
- If total hip replacement becomes necessary in future, the arthroplasty surgical technique will be easier because of:
  - Less incisional and soft-tissue scarring
  - Less hardware to remove or avoid while placing the acetabular components

Overall, studies involving ORIF of osteoporotic fractures using modern techniques (either extensile or minimally invasive) have reported respectable outcomes; however, concerns remain.

- These patients often have multiple comorbidities and are less able to tolerate the significant physiologic insult of the surgery.
- Good fixation in osteoporotic bones is unpredictable.[52]
- Generalized fracture healing in osteoporotic bone has been demonstrated to be impaired in multiple models.[45,53]
- Plate-and-screw constructs are more susceptible to implant failure in osteoporotic bone than in regular bone.[54]
- Despite the observance that elderly patients are more apt than younger patients to tolerate malreduction, several investigators have demonstrated a strong correlation between a worse quality of initial reduction and the incidence of early conversion to THA after geriatric acetabular fractures.[5,27,49]
- Failed treatment with ORIF, which can be in the form of acute fixation failure, early

development of arthritis, or simply persistent pain, can have a large negative impact on functionality and quality of life.

Acute Total Hip Arthroplasty

THA is widely successful in the geriatric population for a variety of conditions, in particular osteoarthritis and femoral neck fractures.[55–58] A significant proportion of geriatric acetabular fracture patients will require eventual conversion to THA. Several investigators have described this rate as between 25% to 31% within 2.4 years after fracture fixation, regardless of the technique used.[5,15,19,20,26,41,48,49] Because a large proportion of geriatric acetabular fracture patients will need THA, it is an attractive idea to perform a single operation to restore maximum functionality as soon as possible. An acute THA in the setting of an unstable acetabular fracture can be a demanding procedure requiring subspecialty expertise in both pelvic trauma and complex arthroplasty techniques. Long operative times are the norm, and the potential for severe complications exists.[59–62]

Acute THA for a geriatric acetabular fracture should be thought of as 2 procedures carried out during the same operative setting. The term "combined hip procedure" was coined to capture this concept.[60] The first stage of the operation involves open reduction and stabilization of the acetabular fracture. Although exact reduction of the articular surface is not necessary, stable support for the acetabular arthroplasty component is an absolute requirement. The columns and walls of the acetabulum will usually be displaced and will require the same reduction and buttress-plate support as ORIF without arthroplasty. As a result, open exposure through an ilioinguinal or other anterior exposure is usually required for the most common anterior-posterior hemitransverse fracture types. After appropriate stabilization of the columns of the acetabulum, the second phase of the surgery involves implantation of the hip arthroplasty components. Fracture fixation is facilitated by removal of the femoral head as an initial step, so that the stages are in fact not distinct and constitute a single surgical strategy. Possibly because of the associated soft-tissue injury and extensive dissection, a high rate of complications such as heterotopic bone, dislocation, and early loosening of acetabular components have been reported.[59–63]

No absolute indications exist for an acute arthroplasty in the setting of an acetabular fracture. If a patient has a fracture that carries a reasonable prognosis with standard operative or nonoperative techniques, acute THA is not appropriate.

However, if the patient has an injury with a poor likelihood of successful acetabular reconstruction, an acute arthroplasty may be a reasonable consideration. Negative prognostic factors for ORIF, which would therefore be relative indications for acute THA, include:

- Poor bone quality
- Comminuted fractures, especially with multiple articular fragments
- Articular impaction
- Associated femoral head impaction
- Associated femoral neck fractures
- Preexisting severe hip osteoarthritis

Several techniques used to perform an acute total hip procedure for acetabular fractures have been described.[59–62,64–67] Individualization to the particular fracture configuration and to the particular comfort and experience of the surgeon is required.

The elderly patient in **Fig. 5** suffered a high-energy trauma, which included a highly comminuted fracture dislocation of her hip. Her posterior wall was in multiple fragments, and she had significant acetabular and femoral articular impaction. Her joint could not be reconstructed, so acute THA was chosen as treatment. The procedure was completed through a Kocher-Langenbeck approach. When performing an acute arthroplasty, excellent acetabular exposure can be obtained through this approach. The femoral head was removed in preparation for the arthroplasty, and the need to protect the blood supply in the quadratus femoris was not required. As a result, wide exposure for fracture stabilization and reaming/positioning of the acetabular component was possible. This patient was treated with reduction and buttressing of the posterior wall with arthroplasty reconstruction using uncemented components with supplemental screw fixation (**Fig. 6**). Note the lag-screw fixation that is possible along the corridor of bone above the sciatic notch, which is easily accessible through the large exposure. Ideally column screw fixation is used to stabilize the acetabulum in preparation for replacement.

The common anterior-hemitransverse fracture pattern is seen in the patient in **Fig. 7**. This patient presented after 3 weeks of nonoperative management at another institution. Because of the poor bone quality and delayed presentation, an acute THA was chosen as treatment. A combined hip procedure was done involving a Kocher-Langenbeck posterior exposure with the patient in the lateral position. After osteotomy of the femoral neck and release of the short rotator muscles including the quadratus femoris, there is

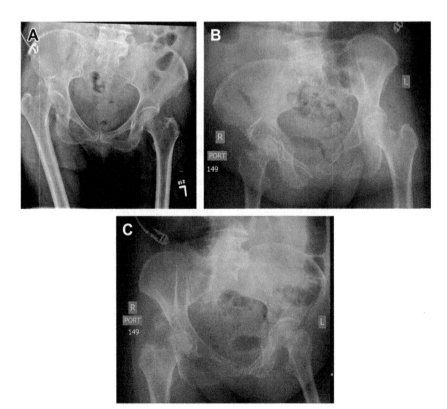

Fig. 5. (*A–C*) Low-energy posterior wall/column fracture dislocation in geriatric patient.

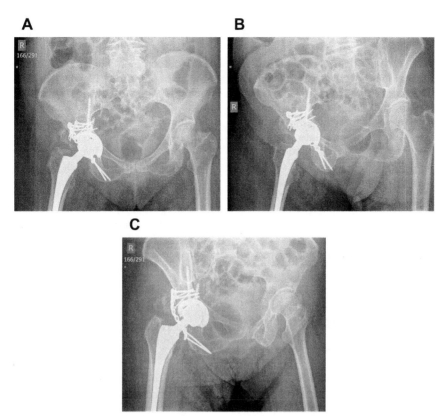

Fig. 6. (A–C) Same patient as in Fig. 5, treated with acute fracture stabilization and THA.

excellent exposure of the posterior column. Stabilization of the quadrilateral plate and anterior column can be achieved with a cabling technique pioneered by Mears and Shirahama.[68] These cables are passed with a long clamp, such as a Kelly clamp, from the posterior approach across the quadrilateral plate, and retrieved near the anterior inferior iliac spine through an iliac crest

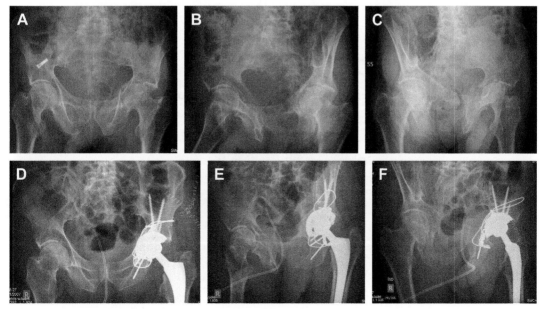

Fig. 7. (A–F) Geriatric acetabular fracture with a "common" anterior-hemitransverse fracture pattern. The patient was treated with combined acute fracture stabilization and THA.

incision. This maneuver gives access similar to the lateral window of an ilioinguinal approach (**Fig. 8**).

These illustrative cases show some available techniques that can be used to stabilize and reconstruct a geriatric acetabular fracture acutely. However, significant technical expertise and long operative times may be required. The medical status of the patient will help to determine whether a prolonged procedure is appropriate. The role of acute THA is controversial, and acetabular trauma surgeons have no consensus on whether it should be routinely offered.[41,42] Because of the potential for significant complications and the morbidity of long surgeries, many investigators recommend a staged arthroplasty approach.

Delayed Total Hip Arthroplasty

Acute arthroplasty is demanding and may be inappropriate for medically compromised patients. Another potential treatment strategy involves arthroplasty as a planned salvage procedure. In this setting, acute management involves ensuring enough bony stability is present to stabilize the acetabular columns and maintain a reduced hip joint, thus allowing early mobilization and sufficient bone healing for successful arthroplasty. In the low-demand elderly patient population, there may be more tolerance for an imperfect reduction during the subacute period while waiting for a THA.

Even if a delayed THA is well planned and well executed, complication rates including infection, dislocation, early loosening, and decreased functional outcome are higher in this setting than with regular primary total hip replacements.[69–72] This finding is expected, given the previously traumatized and often previously operated surgical site. Unfortunately, patients with a failed acetabular fracture have little reconstructive options aside from arthroplasty, so this increased complication rate is accepted. An MIS or limited open procedure that achieves the goals of overall healing of the acetabulum, even without perfect articular reduction, should allow healing of the pelvic columns for restoration of the necessary bone stock required to support an acetabular component. This outcome should decrease the complexity of the delayed arthroplasty. If a patient has a fracture for which nonoperative treatment should allow satisfactory restoration of bone stock, delayed hip arthroplasty need not be preceded by surgery (**Fig. 9**A, B).

To maximize outcome of the delayed arthroplasty:

- A surgeon experienced in complex or post-traumatic arthroplasty is recommended, given the altered anatomy.
- Infection should be ruled out in patients with prior operative fixation using appropriate preoperative workup.

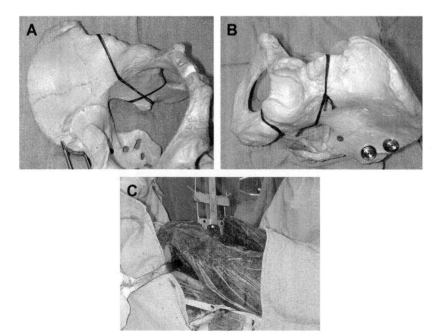

Fig. 8. (*A, B*) Sawbones model of cabling technique. (*C*) Intraoperative photograph demonstrating cable tensioning device and required exposure.

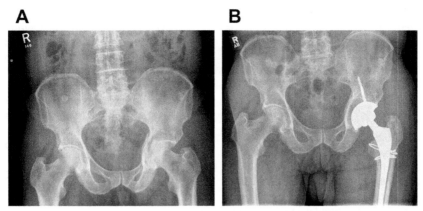

Fig. 9. (*A*) Minimally displaced fracture in patient with multiple comorbidities, poor baseline ambulation status, and inability to comply with protected weight-bearing restrictions. (*B*) After 8 weeks of nonoperative management the patient underwent a planned delayed THA, and returned to fully independent and unaided ambulatory status.

○ Arthroplasty should be staged after a debridement if infection is present
• Only hardware directly interfering with component placement need be removed (**Fig. 10**).

○ High-speed metal-cutting burrs are useful tools for removing obstructive metalwork without extensive dissections
• Acetabular components with screw options are usually required.

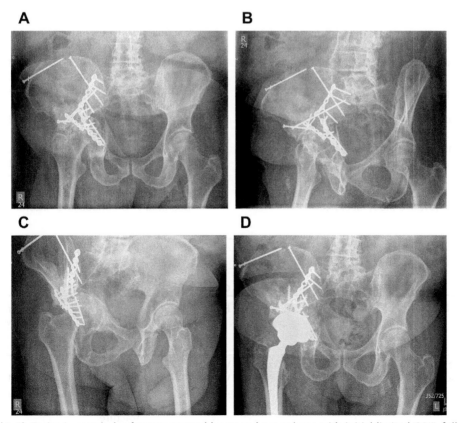

Fig. 10. (*A–D*) Geriatric acetabular fracture treated by staged procedures with initial limited ORIF, followed by arthroplasty 12 weeks later.

- Porous titanium and trabecular metal implants, with or without augments, may be useful.

Prevention of Secondary Fracture

The presence of a fragility fracture is the strongest risk factor for a future fracture, and secondary fractures can have an extremely high associated morbidity and mortality.[9,11,30,73] Therefore, a central goal of the management of any osteoporotic fractures is the prevention of future fractures. While a medical physician usually coordinates pharmacologic management, orthopedic surgeons can greatly improve osteoporosis care.

- Orthopedic surgeons are often the first physician directly involved in the care of a patient with fragility fracture, and thus are obligated to be knowledgable on the management of osteoporosis and facilitate pathways to appropriate care.
- Strategies involving orthopedist-initiated osteoporosis assessment have led to improved access to care, appropriate medication-prescribing practices, compliance, and successful prevention of secondary fracture.[30,33]
- Simply ordering a bone mineral density scan in the orthopedic clinic significantly improves osteoporosis treatment rates by family physicians.[74]

FUTURE RESEARCH AREAS

Compared with the commonly researched fragility fractures in the hip, vertebra, wrist, and humerus, acetabular fragility fractures occur more rarely and are treated by a relatively smaller cohort of surgeons, making research somewhat more difficult. However, this fact also leaves considerable room for innovative study designs.

- A basic but crucial investigation would involve only patients with low-energy acetabular fractures. All current studies on geriatric acetabular fractures are based on age; however, elderly patients make up 9.6% of high-energy orthopedic injuries.[75] A study of only low-energy acetabular fractures is needed to determine the true morbidity and mortality associated with these injuries, rather than confounding the reported numbers with the associated multisystem injuries.
- The current literature pool is also lacking any studies that include nonoperatively treated geriatric acetabular fractures. A recent Cochrane review compared operative with nonoperative management of femoral neck fractures using 5 randomized controlled trials, and concluded that although the incidence of malunion in the nonoperative group was higher, surprisingly there were no significant differences in the rates of nonunion, mortality, long-term pain, or medical complications.[76] It is conceivable that similarly good results could be obtained for patients with acetabular fractures, particularly with minimally displaced fractures. A safe option for non-operative management would improve overall care in at least 2 ways:
  - Enhance access of care, as it would obviate transfer of the patient to a specialized traumatologist or pelvic surgeon
  - Obviate the perceived need to pursue operative management for patients at high surgical risk
- Investigators experienced in this subject have identified a paucity of functional outcome studies on geriatric acetabular fractures.[5,20,26] Decisions regarding which patients are appropriate for MIS fixation rather than acute arthroplasty are not clear, and the inability to accurately prognosticate fracture patterns

Table 1
Care of osteoporotic acetabular fractures

	Nonoperative	MIS	ORIF	Acute ORIF/THR	Delayed THR
Patient factors	Too sick for anesthetic		High demand	Unable to cooperate with restricted weight bearing	Able to mobilize with walking aides
Fracture characteristics	Congruous hip joint	Minimal column displacement	Wall fractures Widely displaced columns	Severe impaction and joint incongruity Femoral head fracture	Minimal impaction/ incongruity

Abbreviations: MIS, minimally invasive surgery; ORIF, open reduction and internal fixation; THR, total hip replacement.

with outcomes can only be solved by larger studies using unbiased recruitment designs and long-term follow-up.

SUMMARY

Fractures of the acetabulum are some of the most challenging fractures that face orthopedic surgeons. In geriatric patients, these challenges are enhanced by the complexity of fracture patterns, the poor biomechanical characteristics of osteoporotic bone, and the comorbidities present in this population. The overriding goals of treatment that must be kept in mind include early mobilization and pain control, optimization of early and later hip-joint function, and minimization of complications from surgical or nonsurgical treatment. Nonoperative care must never consist of prolonged bed rest or traction. Nonsurgical management is preferable when the fracture is stable enough to allow mobilization and healing in a functional position can be expected (**Table 1**).

Operative management is preferred in most patients when significant displacement and/or hip instability are present. ORIF with standard open approaches allows the possibility of an anatomic reduction, and is preferred when the patient can tolerate the necessary surgical insult. Minimally invasive or limited-goals ORIF is an option to restore approximate anatomy and to provide a stable hip and bone stock for future THA. This approach may be appropriate when the patient cannot tolerate a long operation or when fracture characteristics make an anatomic reduction impossible. Acute THA at the time of fracture fixation has a role in select elderly acetabular fractures; however, this combined procedure is associated with long operative sessions, and severe complications can be encountered.

Delayed total hip replacement after acetabular fractures can be successful but is very challenging in the face of significant pelvic nonunion or malunion. If limited ORIF or nonoperative management is chosen initially, the goals of this phase will be to allow early mobilization and reliable healing of the anterior and posterior acetabular columns; this will provide acetabular bone stock for the delayed arthroplasty.

Patients with fragility acetabular fractures have a large number of considerations in play. Patient characteristics determine suitability for operative procedures and functional goals, whereas bone quality and other injury characteristics determine whether an anatomic reconstruction is even feasible. The available expertise of the treating orthopedic surgeon and their institution will also determine what treatment options are safe and available. An individualized plan of care for each patient is necessary taking these factors into account to guide appropriate decision-making and optimize outcomes for patients with these difficult injuries.

REFERENCES

1. Judet R, Judet J, Letournel E. Fractures of the acetabulum: classification and surgical approaches for open reduction. Preliminary report. J Bone Joint Surg Am 1964;46:1615–46.
2. Mears DC. Surgical treatment of acetabular fractures in elderly patients with osteoporotic bone. J Am Acad Orthop Surg 1999;7:128–41.
3. Asadi-Lari M, Tamburini M, Gray D. Patients' needs, satisfaction, and health related quality of life: towards a comprehensive model. Health Qual Life Outcomes 2004;2:32.
4. Harper CM, Lyles YM. Physiology and complications of bed rest. J Am Geriatr Soc 1988;36:1047–54.
5. Helfet DL, Borrelli J Jr, DiPasquale T, et al. Stabilization of acetabular fractures in elderly patients. J Bone Joint Surg Am 1992;74:753–65.
6. Moed BR, McMichael JC. Outcomes of posterior wall fractures of the acetabulum. J Bone Joint Surg Am 2007;89:1170–6.
7. Treatment to prevent osteoporotic fractures: an update. Comparative effectiveness review summary guides for clinicians. Rockville MD. 2007. Available from: http://www.ncbi.nlm.nih.gov/books/NBK43420.
8. Cranney A, Guyatt G, Griffith L, et al. Meta-analyses of therapies for postmenopausal osteoporosis. IX: summary of meta-analyses of therapies for postmenopausal osteoporosis. Endocr Rev 2002;23:570–8.
9. Dell R, Greene D, Schelkun SR, et al. Osteoporosis disease management: the role of the orthopaedic surgeon. J Bone Joint Surg Am 2008;90(Suppl 4): 188–94.
10. Ioannidis G, Papaioannou A, Hopman WM, et al. Relation between fractures and mortality: results from the Canadian Multicentre Osteoporosis Study. CMAJ 2009;181:265–71.
11. Kanis JA. New osteoporosis guidelines for Canada. CMAJ 2010;182:1829–30.
12. Lin JT, Lane JM. Osteoporosis: a review. Clin Orthop Relat Res 2004;126–34.
13. Rossouw JE, Anderson GL, Prentice RL, et al. Risks and benefits of estrogen plus progestin in healthy postmenopausal women: principal results From the Women's Health Initiative randomized controlled trial. JAMA 2002;288:321–33.
14. Sambrook P, Cooper C. Osteoporosis. Lancet 2006; 367:2010–8.
15. Carroll EA, Huber FG, Goldman AT, et al. Treatment of acetabular fractures in an older population. J Orthop Trauma 2010;24:637–44.

16. Johanson NA, Litrenta J, Zampini JM, et al. Surgical treatment options in patients with impaired bone quality. Clin Orthop Relat Res 2011;469:2237–47.

17. World Health Organization. Guidelines for preclinical evaluation and clinical trials in osteoporosis. Geneva (Switzerland): World Health Organization; 1998. p. vi, 68.

18. Abrahamsen B, van Staa T, Ariely R, et al. Excess mortality following hip fracture: a systematic epidemiological review. Osteoporos Int 2009;20:1633–50.

19. Anglen JO, Burd TA, Hendricks KJ, et al. The "gull sign": a harbinger of failure for internal fixation of geriatric acetabular fractures. J Orthop Trauma 2003;17:625–34.

20. Gary JL, VanHal M, Gibbons SD, et al. Functional outcomes in elderly patients with acetabular fractures treated with minimally invasive reduction and percutaneous fixation. J Orthop Trauma 2012;26:278–83.

21. Ferguson TA, Patel R, Bhandari M, et al. Fractures of the acetabulum in patients aged 60 years and older: an epidemiological and radiological study. J Bone Joint Surg Br 2010;92:250–7.

22. Vanderschot P. Treatment options of pelvic and acetabular fractures in patients with osteoporotic bone. Injury 2007;38:497–508.

23. Zelle BA, Cole PA. Open reduction and internal fixation of complex geriatric acetabular fracture. Operat Tech Orthop 2011;21:286–92.

24. Culemann U, Holstein JH, Kohler D, et al. Different stabilisation techniques for typical acetabular fractures in the elderly—a biomechanical assessment. Injury 2010;41:405–10.

25. Hessmann MH, Nijs S, Rommens PM. Acetabular fractures in the elderly. Results of a sophisticated treatment concept. Unfallchirurg 2002;105:893–900 [in German].

26. Jeffcoat DM, Carroll EA, Huber FG, et al. Operative treatment of acetabular fractures in an older population through a limited ilioinguinal approach. J Orthop Trauma 2012;26:284–9.

27. Laflamme GY, Hebert-Davies J, Rouleau D, et al. Internal fixation of osteopenic acetabular fractures involving the quadrilateral plate. Injury 2011;42:1130–4.

28. Cornell CN. Management of acetabular fractures in the elderly patient. HSS J 2005;1:25–30.

29. Pagenkopf E, Grose A, Partal G, et al. Acetabular fractures in the elderly: treatment recommendations. HSS J 2006;2:161–71.

30. Edwards BJ, Koval K, Bunta AD, et al. Addressing secondary prevention of osteoporosis in fracture care: follow-up to "own the bone". J Bone Joint Surg Am 2011;93:e87.

31. Marsh D, Akesson K, Beaton DE, et al. Coordinator-based systems for secondary prevention in fragility fracture patients. Osteoporos Int 2011;22:2051–65.

32. Sale JE, Beaton D, Posen J, et al. Systematic review on interventions to improve osteoporosis investigation and treatment in fragility fracture patients. Osteoporos Int 2011;22:2067–82.

33. Tosi LL, Gliklich R, Kannan K, et al. The American Orthopaedic Association's "own the bone" initiative to prevent secondary fractures. J Bone Joint Surg Am 2008;90:163–73.

34. Letournel É, Judet R, Elson R. Fractures of the acetabulum. 2nd edition. Berlin, New York: Springer-Verlag; 1993. p. xxiii, 733.

35. Matta JM, Anderson LM, Epstein HC, et al. Fractures of the acetabulum. A retrospective analysis. Clin Orthop Relat Res 1986;230–40.

36. Spencer RF. Acetabular fractures in older patients. J Bone Joint Surg Br 1989;71:774–6.

37. Arora R, Lutz M, Deml C, et al. A prospective randomized trial comparing nonoperative treatment with volar locking plate fixation for displaced and unstable distal radial fractures in patients sixty-five years of age and older. J Bone Joint Surg Am 2011;93:2146–53.

38. Court-Brown CM, Garg A, McQueen MM. The translated two-part fracture of the proximal humerus. Epidemiology and outcome in the older patient. J Bone Joint Surg Br 2001;83:799–804.

39. Zyto K. Non-operative treatment of comminuted fractures of the proximal humerus in elderly patients. Injury 1998;29:349–52.

40. Karpman RR, Del Mar NB. Supracondylar femoral fractures in the frail elderly. Fractures in need of treatment. Clin Orthop Relat Res 1995;21–4.

41. Kreder HJ, Rozen N, Borkhoff CM, et al. Determinants of functional outcome after simple and complex acetabular fractures involving the posterior wall. J Bone Joint Surg Br 2006;88(6):776–82.

42. Pohlemann T, Culemann U. Summary of controversial debates during the 5th "Homburg Pelvic Course" 13-15 September 2006. Injury 2007;38:424–30.

43. Siska PA. Treatment of low-energy geriatric acetabular fractures with protrusion. Operat Tech Orthop 2011;21:276–9.

44. Silver JJ, Einhorn TA. Osteoporosis and aging. Current update. Clin Orthop Relat Res 1995;10–20.

45. Cornell CN, Ayalon O. Evidence for success with locking plates for fragility fractures. HSS J 2011;7:164–9.

46. Ekeland A, Engesoeter LB, Langeland N. Influence of age on mechanical properties of healing fractures and intact bones in rats. Acta Orthop Scand 1982;53:527–34.

47. Sands SS, Sagi HC. Open reduction of geriatric acetabulum fractures using a Stoppa exposure. Operat Tech Orthop 2011;21:272–5.

48. Starr AJ, Jones AL, Reinert CM, et al. Preliminary results and complications following limited open

reduction and percutaneous screw fixation of displaced fractures of the acetabulum. Injury 2001; 32(Suppl 1):SA45–50.

49. Gary JL, Lefaivre KA, Gerold F, et al. Survivorship of the native hip joint after percutaneous repair of acetabular fractures in the elderly. Injury 2011;42: 1144–51.

50. Kim YH, Kim JS, Park JW, et al. Comparison of total hip replacement with and without cement in patients younger than 50 years of age: the results at 18 years. J Bone Joint Surg Br 2011;93:449–55.

51. Polkowski GG, Callaghan JJ, Mont MA, et al. Total hip arthroplasty in the very young patient. J Am Acad Orthop Surg 2012;20:487–97.

52. Cornell CN. Internal fracture fixation in patients with osteoporosis. J Am Acad Orthop Surg 2003;11: 109–19.

53. Borrelli J Jr, Pape C, Hak D, et al. Physiological challenges of bone repair. J Orthop Trauma 2012;26: 708–11.

54. Giannoudis PV, Schneider E. Principles of fixation of osteoporotic fractures. J Bone Joint Surg Br 2006; 88:1272–8.

55. Boettcher WG. Total hip arthroplasties in the elderly. Morbidity, mortality, and cost effectiveness. Clin Orthop Relat Res 1992;30–4.

56. Pagnano MW, Levy BA, Berry DJ. Cemented all polyethylene tibial components in patients age 75 years and older. Clin Orthop Relat Res 1999;73–80.

57. Shah AK, Celestin J, Parks ML, et al. Long-term results of total joint arthroplasty in elderly patients who are frail. Clin Orthop Relat Res 2004;106–9.

58. Zi-Sheng A, You-Shui G, Zhi-Zhen J, et al. Hemiarthroplasty vs primary total hip arthroplasty for displaced fractures of the femoral neck in the elderly: a meta-analysis. J Arthroplasty 2012;27:583–90.

59. Boraiah S, Ragsdale M, Achor T, et al. Open reduction internal fixation and primary total hip arthroplasty of selected acetabular fractures. J Orthop Trauma 2009;23:243–8.

60. Herscovici D Jr, Lindvall E, Bolhofner B, et al. The combined hip procedure: open reduction internal fixation combined with total hip arthroplasty for the management of acetabular fractures in the elderly. J Orthop Trauma 2010;24:291–6.

61. Joly MJ, Mears DC. The role of total hip arthroplasty in acetabular fracture management. Operat Tech Orthop 1993;3:80–102.

62. Mears DC, Velyvis JH. Acute total hip arthroplasty for selected displaced acetabular fractures: two to twelve-year results. J Bone Joint Surg Am 2002;84: 1–9.

63. Sarkar MR, Wachter N, Kinzl L, et al. Acute total hip replacement for displaced acetabular fractures in older patients. Eur J Trauma 2004;30:296–304.

64. Marcantonio AJ, Iorio R, Specht LM, et al. Acute total hip replacement combined with open reduction internal fixation (ORIF) for the management of acetabular fracture in the elderly. Operat Tech Orthop 2011;21:293–7.

65. Mears DC, Velyvis JH. Primary total hip arthroplasty after acetabular fracture. Instr Course Lect 2001;50: 335–54.

66. Mouhsine E, Garofalo R, Borens O, et al. Cable fixation and early total hip arthroplasty in the treatment of acetabular fractures in elderly patients. J Arthroplasty 2004;19:344–8.

67. Beaule PE, Griffin DB, Matta JM. The Levine anterior approach for total hip replacement as the treatment for an acute acetabular fracture. J Orthop Trauma 2004;18:623–9.

68. Mears DC, Shirahama M. Stabilization of an acetabular fracture with cables for acute total hip arthroplasty. J Arthroplasty 1998;13:104–7.

69. Bellabarba C, Berger RA, Bentley CD, et al. Cementless acetabular reconstruction after acetabular fracture. J Bone Joint Surg Am 2001;83:868–76.

70. Ranawat A, Zelken J, Helfet D, et al. Total hip arthroplasty for posttraumatic arthritis after acetabular fracture. J Arthroplasty 2009;24:759–67.

71. Sermon A, Broos P, Vanderschot P. Total hip replacement for acetabular fractures. Results in 121 patients operated between 1983 and 2003. Injury 2008;39:914–21.

72. Chen AF, McClain EJ, Klatt BA. Delayed total hip replacement for posttraumatic arthritis in the geriatric patient after fractured acetabulum. Operat Tech Orthop 2011;21:298–305.

73. Adler RA. Secondary fracture prevention. Curr Osteoporos Rep 2012;10:22–7.

74. Rozental TD, Makhni EC, Day CS, et al. Improving evaluation and treatment for osteoporosis following distal radial fractures. A prospective randomized intervention. J Bone Joint Surg Am 2008;90:953–61.

75. Keller JM, Sciadini MF, Sinclair E, et al. Geriatric trauma: demographics, injuries, and mortality. J Orthop Trauma 2012;26:e161–5.

76. Handoll HH, Parker MJ. Conservative versus operative treatment for hip fractures in adults. Cochrane Database Syst Rev 2008;(3):CD000337.

Osteoporotic Pelvic Ring Injuries

Michael P. Leslie, DO*, Michael R. Baumgaertner, MD

KEYWORDS

- Osteoporotic pelvic fractures • Lateral compression • External fixation • Transsacral screw fixation
- Early mobilization

KEY POINTS

- Osteoporotic pelvic ring injuries have historically been treated nonoperatively.
- Osteoporotic patients are not only elderly, and continue to be active and demanding of a return to ambulatory lifestyles.
- Injuries need to be delineated as high-energy versus low-energy.
- The implications of injury patterns may be quite different for osteoporotic patients, as ligamentous structures rarely are included as part of their injury spectrum.
- Treatment options vary greatly from those typically chosen for young patients.

INCIDENCE

The osteoporotic pelvic ring injury is grossly underrepresented in the reporting of all pelvic ring injuries. Historically most of these injuries were treated nonoperatively, with little attention paid to the individual fracture pattern. The combination of an increasing geriatric population with greater demands for function, and their complex medical comorbidities, makes pelvic ring injuries a life-changing event for each patient. In North America there are no published estimates of the incidence of osteoporotic pelvic ring injuries. Overall the incidence of pelvic ring fractures varies from 0.3% to 8% of all fractures.[1] The force needed to impart a pelvic ring fracture has been estimated at 2000 to 10,000 N on nonosteoporotic bone.[2] This premise alludes to 2 important points: (1) if a high-energy force is delivered to osteoporotic bone, the patient is likely to sustain a significantly worse injury to the soft tissues; and (2) the increasing incidence of pelvic trauma in osteoporotic patients is not secondary to high-energy trauma.

In Finland, from 1970 to 1997 there was a 23% increase in the age-adjusted incidence of pelvic ring in combination with a 6-year increase in the median age of the patients suffering these fractures.[3] This long-term population study suggested that the number of osteoporotic pelvic ring fractures could triple by the year 2030. If this trend is extrapolated to a worldwide estimation, in those countries where osteoporosis is highly prevalent the number of pelvic ring injuries will be staggering. This study also elucidates that the large preponderance of these fractures (83%) was due to a ground-level fall secondary to a multifactorial gait disturbance. This fact needs to be considered in the context of the acute increase, since that time, in numbers of geriatric patients who continue to live active lives (including driving), which will clearly lead to an increase in the incidence of high-energy pelvic ring injuries in parallel with low-energy fractures of the pelvis. Overall this incidence should be reflected in a much more commonly studied fracture, that of proximal femoral fractures (hip fractures). There has in fact

Disclosures: None.
Conflicts of Interest: None.
Department of Orthopaedics and Rehabilitation, Yale University School of Medicine, PO Box 208071, New Haven, CT 06520-8071, USA
* Corresponding author.
E-mail address: Michael.leslie@yale.edu

Orthop Clin N Am 44 (2013) 217–224
http://dx.doi.org/10.1016/j.ocl.2013.01.007
0030-5898/13/$ – see front matter © 2013 Elsevier Inc. All rights reserved.

orthopedic.theclinics.com

been a significant decrease in the overall incidence of hip fractures in the period from 1995 to 2005 according to Medicare databases, with a decline of 24.5% in women 19.2% in men. The suspected cause of the decline is the use of bisphosphonate therapy, and this is a critical finding in these patients, as the number of their comorbid medical conditions continues to increase.[4] It is unknown whether the incidence of pelvic ring fractures is following that of hip fractures; however, it is clear that, similar to the history of hip fracture treatment, the techniques of fixation and rehabilitation needed for osteoporotic pelvic ring injuries must evolve to meet patients' expectations for an active lifestyle, much as they have for patients with osteoporotic proximal femur fracture.

ANATOMY

Pelvic anatomy is composed of innominate and sacral bones along with soft-tissue attachments that, on fracture, act to both stabilize and potentially displace the skeleton. In young patients, low-energy injuries typically result in purely soft-tissue injuries, and osseous injuries are often bony avulsions. In the elderly patient, the bony anatomy typically fails with minimal trauma and the soft tissues (ligaments) rarely fail in significant fashion. Therefore, remarkable fractures of the osteoporotic pelvis may not be markedly unstable. The primary ligaments in the pelvis include the sacrotuberous, sacrospinous, anterior sacroiliac, and posterior sacroiliac. Additional constraints include the pubic symphysis and the iliolumbar ligaments. The vascular anatomy is often calcified as well as compromised in the geriatric osteoporotic patient. This finding may be a harbinger of poor healing capacity that should be considered when directing any potential surgical intervention. Urologic injury is estimated to be present in 15% to 45% of all pelvic ring injuries, but this is typically confined to high-energy lateral compression and anteroposterior compression injuries. All of these issues must be considered in planning treatment.

EVALUATION OF THE PATIENT WITH OSTEOPOROTIC PELVIC TRAUMA
Mechanism of Injury

The large majority of osteoporotic pelvic ring injuries result from low-energy mechanisms; however, this should not be assumed. With the increased incidence of older patients driving and working, the possibility arises that their trauma is the result of high energy. A careful history along with a description of the scene and understanding of any other injuries that may have occurred to other patients are key considerations.

Low-Energy Pelvic Ring Injuries

A fall from a standing position is the most common mechanism for an osteoporotic patient presenting with a pelvic ring injury. Often these patients are unable to ambulate and are evaluated in an emergency department setting. A careful history and physical examination is paramount. These patients may present with marked dementia and are unable to effectively communicate. In addition, they might suffer from medical conditions that predispose them to bony injury. For example, the growing population with rheumatoid arthritis incurs a 1.5-times higher rate of fracture than age-matched controls.[5] This history may also influence the decision-making tree in treatment, as patients may be on medications that can interfere with wound healing and anesthesia. Some critical points in the medical history that deserve special consideration include a history of malignancy in the pelvis requiring radiation, a history of surgery in the lumbar spine requiring dorsal bone grafting, and a history of treatment for osteoporosis.[6]

A complete physical examination should include a focused neurologic evaluation, as comminuted fractures of the posterior pelvic ring often will injure the exiting nerve roots to varying degrees. In addition, a careful evaluation of the skin is required, as disruption may occur owing to poor quality, as well as a clinical evaluation of leg length. Radiographic evaluation should begin with an anteroposterior view of the pelvis. The most common findings of fracture on this image will be of the superior and inferior pubic ramus. The constellation of rami fractures along with their individual orientation may predict potential displacement, which should elicit further evaluation with inlet and outlet radiographs, computed tomography (CT) imaging, or both. The latter is particularly important for evaluation of the posterior pelvic ring, where it is estimated that 30% of pelvic ring injuries are missed without the combination of both CT and plain radiography.[7] The most common bony injury in the posterior pelvis is a fracture of the sacrum lateral to the foramina and medial to the sacroiliac joint. This fracture line is usually incomplete, but should be examined on the coronal CT format to determine if the fracture indeed exits the posterior sacrum. The key point in radiographic evaluation, however, is that there is rarely injury to the pelvic ligaments in osteoporotic patients because the strength of these ligaments exceeds that of the osteoporotic pelvic bone. As such, a severe bony injury from a low-energy mechanism may be stable and does not warrant surgical intervention. Recognition of potential bilateral vertical sacral fractures connected through disc spaces or vertebral bodies, which will often occur through a severely degenerated region of the bone, can change treatment recommendations significantly. These fractures may represent the high-energy variant in young patients known as spinopelvic dissociation.[6] In addition, evaluation of the lumbar spine and pelvic ring for periprosthetic fractures in the presence of existing hardware can be accomplished by CT. Examples might include disruption of a pedicle around a screw placed during a prior lumbar fusion procedure, or a periprosthetic acetabular fracture around a pubic root fracture. Discovery of such injuries may affect surgical planning.

A more complex group of patients with low-energy pelvic ring fracture are those with suspected altered biomechanics attributable to a myriad of causes that essentially allow for insufficiency fractures, particularly of the sacrum but also of the rami. Often these fractures are discovered accidentally, and the risk factors identified have included osteoporosis, rheumatoid arthritis, corticosteroid treatment, and mechanical constraint from prior instrumentation.[8] These fractures are often not identified immediately, and a delay in diagnosis can range from 1 to 3 months. Magnetic resonance imaging in a patient with negative physical and plain radiography findings, but recalcitrant low back pain, may yield the diagnosis and allow for careful treatment.

Treatment of low-energy fractures

The patient with low-energy pelvic fracture may have a radiograph with fracture patterns that appear to fit into the Young and Burgess or the Tile classification systems, but the treatment varies widely because the mechanisms do not impart nearly the same energy into the pelvic ring.[2,9] Therefore, the classification of these injuries in the same systems used for high-energy fracture is questionable. Hemodynamic instability secondary to the fracture is also rarely present on presentation, so the use of pelvic binders, sheets, C-clamps, and external fixators is rarely indicated. In fact the use of a C-clamp may be directly contraindicated by the insufficiency of the posterior pelvis in avoiding iatrogenic injury.

The tenet of treatment for all osteoporotic fractures is early mobilization. It is well known that extended periods of bed rest will lead to pneumonia, decubitus ulceration, deep venous thrombosis and, in the case of the pelvis, will often not lead to avoidance of a subsequent deformity.

This evidence is extrapolated from data on fractures of the proximal femur, for which early mobilization has become the gold standard.

Ideally the patient should be treated with minimized weight bearing with an assistive device on the affected side. Given their advanced age and risk for falls, many osteoporotic patients are maintained as weight bearing as tolerated, with appropriate analgesics and venothromboembolic prophylaxis (pharmacologic and mechanical). Some authors have recommended postmobilization imaging to visualize fractures that potentially might not have been easily visualized on initial radiographs or even CT, owing to the marked osteoporotic changes (**Fig. 1**).[6] If patients are unable to mobilize effectively for reasons of pain control, it has been postulated that compression of the posterior pelvic ring (sacral fracture) can lead to decreased pain and increased ambulatory capacity.[10] The relative osteoporotic sacral vertebral bodies do not contain bone stock adequate enough to achieve compression across the sacral fracture, therefore the use of long-screw fixation known as transsacral screw fixation, which traverses the entire sacrum and engages the contralateral ilium, is recommended. This type of fixation is technically demanding and requires familiarity with the technique so as to avoid iatrogenic injury to neurovascular structures.[11] Alternatively, if the fracture is contained to zone I of the sacrum and is nondisplaced, there is growing support for the use of sacroplasty whereby bone cement is injected percutaneously into the region of the fracture to fill in the defect created by the fracture. Significant pain relief is noted, similar to vertebroplasty, and the opportunity to augment the cement with iliosacral or transsacral screw fixation remains a viable option.[12] A question that has not been answered is whether the use of calcium phosphate or calcium sulfate bone substitutes in this region would provide improved incorporation and the ability to insert screws for fixation rather than cement.

Treatment of the anterior pelvic ring in the low-energy fracture pattern rarely requires open operative reduction and plate stabilization, but patients may benefit from anterior ring distraction by either internal or external devices that can be applied through the supra-acetabular corridor. This type of treatment may effectively reduce the risk of internal rotation. The difficulty with these techniques is the inability of achieving adequate intraoperative imaging in a markedly osteoporotic patient.

Complications of nonoperative care include the risk of pelvic deformity, including internal rotation and hemipelvic flexion deformity; however, such

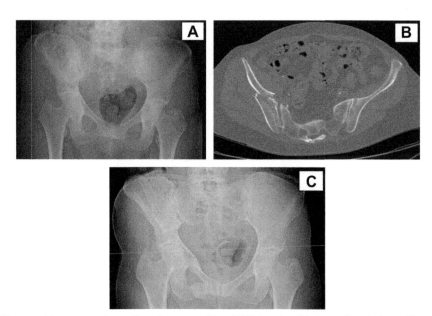

Fig. 1. An 86-year-old woman who suffered a ground-level fall in a local bakery. (*A, B*) She suffered a complex lateral compression injury with a comminuted intra-articular posterior ilium fracture and ipsilateral displaced superior and inferior pubic rami fractures. After extensive discussion, she was able to mobilize and chose nonoperative care. (*C*) Moderate deformity at full bony healing 1 year after injury. She experiences no pain, and wears a shoe lift for her clinically relevant leg-length discrepancy and internal rotation deformity.

deformity is well tolerated by most patients of advanced age. The risk of nonunion at any part of the pelvic ring is unclear, particularly in low-energy fractures in the elderly. There are numerous reports of pelvic ring nonunion in the literature, most of which concern patients with high-energy injuries who are inadequately treated. The low rate of pelvic nonunion is attributed to adequate blood supply and a large surface area of cancellous bone.[13] When nonunion occurs, treatment recommendations include take-down of atrophic nonunions and plate stabilization, or retrograde intramedullary screw compression using multiplanar fluoroscopy for hypertrophic nonunions. There are no data regarding the rate of nonunion of the osteoporotic pelvis.

Insufficiency Fracture Due to Malignancy or Radiation

There is a subset of pelvic fractures that often do not involve any evidence of trauma, and many of these patients report waking up with acute pain in the groin or overlying the ischial tuberosity when sitting. Extensive literature documents the risk of both metastatic lesions and postradiation osteonecrosis in the pathogenesis of fracture. In one study, the risk of atraumatic pelvic fracture following pelvic irradiation for all types of gynecologic malignancies was 11.4% within 6 months.[14] The treatment modalities used for osteoporotic

fractures are often challenged by poor bone quality, and the focus of treatment should be on analgesia, restricted weight bearing, and reduction of radiation dose to areas of the bone at particular risk of fracture, including the sacral ala and the rami, without compromising the radiation dose needed for tumor control. Surgical treatment can be difficult in these patients, and augmentation of the bone might be necessary (**Fig. 2**).

High-Energy Injury

With the increasing activity level of elderly patients in conjunction with the occurrence of osteoporosis in younger patients, the incidence of high-energy displaced fractures is on the increase. These fractures fit more precisely into the familiar mechanistic and anatomic classification schemes with which most orthopedists are familiar.[2,9] The outcomes of nonoperative care of unstable pelvic ring injuries have been consistently reported as dismal in all series of young patients. In Tile type B and type C injuries, Fell and colleagues[15] reported 55% and 85% residual pain, respectively. In addition, a 90% functional deficit was reported in type C injuries. Considering the overall debilitating effects of the fractures in young patients, if the osteoporotic fracture occurs as a result of a high-energy mechanism, attention to detail and treatment according to the principles of internal fixation should be undertaken (**Fig. 3**).

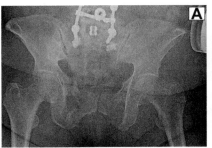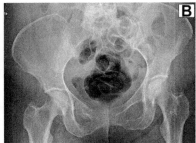

Fig. 2. Fractures suffered in markedly osteoporotic patients. (*A*) A 75-year-old woman with atraumatic multiple fragility fractures years after multiple spine surgeries including L4-S1 arthrodesis with augmentation in the sacrum. (*B*) A 45-year-old woman who recently suffered her 13th fragility fracture in her pelvis, with rami fractures on the right (no posterior ring injury).

Lateral compression injuries comprise the large majority of pelvic ring injuries in the osteoporotic population. As a result, the anterior pelvic ring is often a simple oblique or comminuted fracture of the superior and inferior ramus. With this injury pattern an injury to the bladder or other visceral organ can occur, but vascular injury is rare because the deforming force is internal rotation. The posterior pelvic ring is of particular importance in considering treatment. In young patients the fracture is most commonly a disruption of the sacroiliac joint, or a zone II sacral fracture with displacement. The osteoporotic patient may more commonly suffer an iliac fracture that extends into the sacroiliac joint. This fracture should be carefully mapped out such that the level of fracture in relation to the sacral vertebral bodies can be re-established if possible. Many lateral compression injuries lead to fracture patterns that are consistent with vertically unstable fracture patterns, which

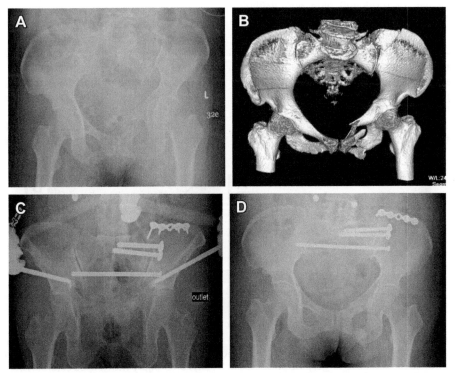

Fig. 3. (*A–D*) An 81 year-old woman, struck by a motor vehicle, who suffered lateral compression type II injury. She was treated in skeletal traction until postinjury day 16, when she was physiologically ready to undergo open reduction internal fixation. Surgical reduction included restoration of her extra-articular iliac segment, which was then stabilized with iliosacral screw fixation, and reinforced with transsacral screw fixation at S2 and anterior ring external fixation for 8 weeks.

can lead to leg-length discrepancy and rotational deformity that might only be acceptable to a medically infirm patient.

To achieve early mobilization and avoid complications such as nonunion and pelvic deformity with associated leg-length discrepancy, it is important to carefully plan surgical intervention. This planning must come with an understanding that reduction aids, such as Schanz pins in the medius tubercle and pelvic reduction clamps, may not function as effectively owing to the insufficiency of the underlying bone. These reduction aids incur a risk of bony cutout and eventual compromise of the definitive fixation surfaces. In addition, no devices have been specifically designed for the fixation of osteoporotic pelvic bone. The principles that must be considered are consistent with those of standard implants applied using techniques specific to the bone quality of each patient (**Fig. 4**).

FIXATION OPTIONS FOR OSTEOPOROTIC FRACTURES

When a displaced pelvic ring injury occurs in an osteoporotic patient, often focus of treatment is less on emergent stabilization and more on the unique use of reduction aids and fixation modalities.

Anterior Pelvic Ring

Historically the fixation of the anterior ring has been solely through external fixation to both the iliac wing and/or the supra-acetabular corridor. External fixators are fraught with difficulties, including patient dissatisfaction, and the inability to maintain the pins for an extended period of time owing to infection and pin loosening has brought the utility of this treatment into question. Some of the newest advances have been in the type of pin used, for example, hydroxyapatite-coated pins, which promote bone ingrowth and therefore decrease pin loosening. Other techniques of stabilizing the anterior pelvic ring include internal fixation that spans both hemipelvises. This outcome can be achieved through the use of contoured pelvic reconstruction plates that span both sides of the pelvis and allow the use of locking-screw fixation and long-screw fixation in the posterior column. An additional technique that has been described for the anterior pelvic ring is the use of a retrograde intramedullary screw for the superior pubic ramus, particularly for hypertrophic nonunion that requires increased stability.[16]

Posterior Pelvic Ring

As discussed earlier, posterior pelvic ring injury is often quite diverse and requires extensive surgical planning. The focus of instability is the key point to be elucidated, whether this is primarily an intra-articular ilium fracture, sacroiliac joint dislocation, or sacral fracture. If there is a complete sacral fracture with vertical displacement, fixation should be carried out to avoid the vertical shear forces that work across the fracture. This goal is best accomplished by transsacral screw fixation, if possible, and often the S2 corridor may provide a useful level on which to achieve fixation. Fixation is most safely accomplished by achieving as anatomic a reduction as possible, thus creating a safe passageway for intramedullary screw fixation.[17] Often this is best accomplished by reconstructing the extra-articular ilium in similar fashion

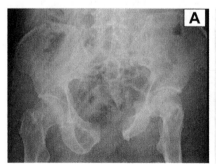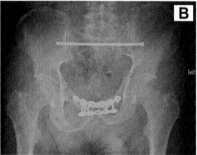

Fig. 4. (*A*, *B*) A 75-year-old man who fell from a ladder in another country, where he was placed into an iliac wing external fixator for 8 days, at which point it was removed and the injury left to deform because he was thought to be too unstable for definitive surgery. He presented at 54 days after injury with a fixed external rotation deformity and a marked leg-length discrepancy. Multiple osteoporotic pelvic ring criteria are appreciated as he underwent a sacral osteotomy, followed by dual plating of his anterior ring and transsacral screw fixation of his comminuted deformed posterior ring. Careful attention was paid to avoid reduction techniques that would compromise his bone stock. Minor leg-length discrepancy was deemed acceptable, and he is pain free and ambulatory 9 months postoperatively.

to open reduction/internal fixation of a crescent fracture. Instead of the primary fixation with plates and intraosseous screws achieved in young patients (anterior column and sciatic buttress screw fixation), transsacral screw fixation can be used in the osteoporotic patient to achieve long screw lengths with better purchase in intact bone. If the sacroiliac joint is unstable, some investigators have advocated primary fusion via an anterior approach with compression, using intramedullary screw fixation or plate and screw fixation.[6] The other, sometimes unappreciated, location of instability is the sacrum, in bilateral vertical fractures that cross the midline or in fractures that disrupt the L5-S1 facet joints on one or both sides (spinal pelvic disassociation). In this case, multilevel transsacral screw fixation or lumbopelvic fixation may be chosen. When an associated spinal injury requiring additional lumbar spine fusion or a preexisting lumbar fusion is present, strong consideration should be given to lumbopelvic fixation. However, in osteoporotic patients this procedure is fraught with difficulty, with problems such as prone positioning in an elderly patient, extensive surgical insult, and hardware prominence.[18]

FUTURE DEVELOPMENTS

Recent publications have suggested the use of a subcutaneous internal fixator that uses polyaxial pedicle screw fixation within the supra-acetabular corridor and a prebent rod inserted outside the fascia.[19] There are many potential advantages to this type of approach in the osteoporotic patient. The sciatic buttress where this pedicle screw engages the bone is typically reliable, and gentle reduction maneuvers can be used with compression or distracting devices. Often this can be used to achieve a reduction, after which posterior percutaneous screw fixation can be performed to compress the sacral fracture. Future developments of this type of treatment may include cement augmentation of the pedicle screw, similar to what is now performed in the pedicles of the spine (**Fig. 5**).

Another unique method of reduction and percutaneous fixation has been described by Matta and Yerasimides[20] for high-energy complete zone II sacral fractures with ipsilateral rami fractures. This method uses an orthopedic specialty table and allows for minimal surgical trauma. Using distal femoral mechanized traction in the prone position with hyperextension at the hip, correction of the flexion deformity can be achieved. This procedure occasionally requires fixation of the intact hemipelvis to the operating-room table and

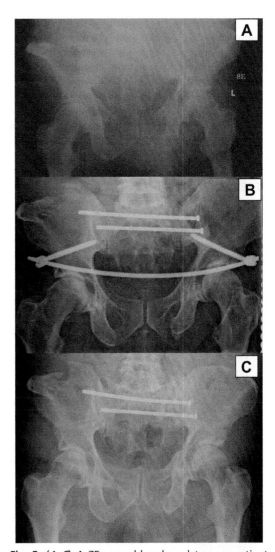

Fig. 5. (A–C) A 75-year-old male polytrauma patient whose pelvis was stabilized with an internal anterior fixator with transsacral screw fixation posteriorly. The anterior ring fixator was removed at 3 months, and 6 months postoperatively he ambulates without assistive device or pain.

external fixation in the prone position to fine-tune the reduction.[20]

SUMMARY

Injuries of the pelvic ring can be devastating high-energy traumatic fractures. With the advancing age of the baby-boomer generation and the increasing number of medical comorbidities that include osteoporosis and also inhibit healthy bony metabolism through polypharmacy, pelvic ring injuries are becoming more common. Careful evaluation of each patient, with delineation of the mechanism and concurrent soft-tissue injuries are paramount in developing a comprehensive treatment plan.[21] As is the case with many osteoporotic fractures, there is no single algorithm that fits each patient. The most critical points to remember are that these patients cannot be treated as young high-energy trauma patients, and that the underlying cause of their fractures may be unrelated to the apparent trauma and may be more integrally related to underlying metabolic problems of the bone or even malignancy.

REFERENCES

1. Fuchs T, Rottbeck U, Hofbauer V, et al. Pelvic ring fractures in the elderly. Underestimated osteoporotic fracture. Unfallchirurg 2011;114:663–70 [in German].
2. Tile M, Hear T, Vrahas M. Biomechanics of the pelvic ring. In: Tile M, Helfet DL, Kellam JF, editors. Fractures of the pelvis and acetabulum. 3rd edition. Philadelphia: Lippincott Williams and Wilkins; 2003. p. 32–45.
3. Kannus P, Palvanen M, Miemi S, et al. Epidemiology of osteoporotic pelvic fractures in elderly people in Finland: sharp increase in 1970-1997 and alarming projections for the new millennium. Osteoporos Int 2000;11:443–8.
4. Brauer CA, Coca-Perraillon M, Cutler DM, et al. Incidence and mortality of hip fractures in the United States. JAMA 2009;302:1573–9.
5. Kim SY, Schneeweiss S, Liu J, et al. Risk of osteoporotic fracture in a large population-based cohort of patients with rheumatoid arthritis. Arthritis Res Ther 2010;12:R154.
6. Rommens PM, Wagner D, Hofmann A. Surgical management of osteoporotic pelvic fractures: a new challenge. Eur J Trauma Emerg Surg 2012;38:499–509.
7. Berg EE, Chebuhar C, Bell RM. Pelvic trauma imaging: a blinded comparison of computed tomography and roentgenograms. J Trauma 1996;41:994–8.
8. Schapira D, Militeanu D, Israel O, et al. Insufficiency fractures of the pubic ramus. Semin Arthritis Rheum 1996;25:373–82.
9. Burgess AR, Eastridge BJ, Young JW, et al. Pelvic ring disruptions: effective classification system and treatment protocols. J Trauma 1990;30:848–56.
10. Barei DP, Shafer BL, Beingessner DM, et al. The impact of open reduction internal fixation on acute pain management in unstable pelvic ring injuries. J Trauma 2010;68:949–53.
11. Gardner MJ, Routt ML Jr. Transiliac-transsacral screws for posterior pelvic stabilization. J Orthop Trauma 2011;25:378–84.
12. Waites MD, Mears SC, Mathis JM, et al. The strength of the osteoporotic sacrum. Spine 2007;32:E652–5.
13. Archdeacon MT, Kuhlman G, Kazemi N. Fellow's corner: grand rounds from the University of Cincinnati Medical Center—painful superior and inferior pubic rami nonunion. J Orthop Trauma 2010;24:e109–12.
14. Ikushima H, Osaki K, Furutani S, et al. Pelvic bone complications following radiation therapy of gynecologic malignancies: clinical evaluation of radiation induced pelvic insufficiency fractures. Gynecol Oncol 2006;103:1100–4.
15. Fell M, Meissner A, Rahmanzadeh R. Long-term outcome after conservative treatment of pelvic ring injuries and conclusions for current management. Zentralbl Chir 1995;120:899–904.
16. Routt ML Jr, Simonian PT, Grujic L. The retrograde medullary superior pubic ramus screw for the treatment of anterior pelvic ring disruptions: a new technique. J Orthop Trauma 1995;9:35–44.
17. Reilly MC, Bono CM, Litkouhi B, et al. The effect of sacral fracture malreduction on the safe placement of iliosacral screws. J Orthop Trauma 2003;17:88–94.
18. Sagi HC. Technical aspects and recommended treatment algorithms in triangular osteosynthesis and spinopelvic fixation for vertical shear transforaminal sacral fractures. J Orthop Trauma 2009;23:354–60.
19. Vaidya R, Colen R, Vigdorchik J, et al. Treatment of unstable pelvic ring injuries with an internal anterior fixator and posterior fixation: initial clinical series. J Orthop Trauma 2012;26:1–8.
20. Matta JM, Yerasimides JG. Table-skeletal fixation as an adjunct to pelvic ring reduction. J Orthop Trauma 2007;21:647–56.
21. Vanderschot P. Treatment options of pelvic and acetabular fractures in patients with osteoporotic bone. Injury 2007;38:497–508.

Osteoporotic Ankle Fractures

Joshua R. Olsen, MD[a],*, Joshua Hunter, MD[a],
Judith F. Baumhauer, MD, MPH[a,b]

KEYWORDS

- Osteoporotic ankle fractures • Elderly • Outcomes • Surgical fixation

KEY POINTS

- Osteoporotic ankle fractures commonly occur in the elderly and are anticipated to increase in incidence over the next 20 years.
- Ankle fractures differ from vertebral and hip fractures in the elderly and are associated with different risk factors.
- The initial assessment of elderly patients with ankle fractures should be thorough and must take into consideration ambulatory status; comorbidities, such as diabetes mellitus; dementia; and bone health.
- Good surgical outcomes are obtained in elderly patients with unstable ankle fractures. Diabetes, peripheral vascular disease, smoking, and dementia have been associated with increased postsurgical complications.
- Several different surgical techniques have been described to achieve stable fixation in patients with osteoporotic ankle fractures with good results.

INTRODUCTION: DEFINING THE PROBLEM

Ankle fractures in the elderly pose a significant burden on society and health care in the United States. Also referred to as low-energy trauma, age-related, or fragility fractures in the literature, ankle fractures are one of the most common fractures in the elderly and its incidence will likely increase over the next 20 years in developed nations.[1–3] Moreover, although their true economic impact is unknown, healthcare costs for osteoporotic ankle fractures is estimated to increase over the next decade as is projected for other fragility fractures.[4]

A concept that has emerged in epidemiologic studies, and at first glance seems counterintuitive, is that osteoporosis is not a risk factor for ankle fractures. In 2003, Hasselman and colleagues[5] followed more than 9000 elderly white women for a 10-year period and documented 291 ankle fractures. Risk factors for ankle fractures in this cohort included younger age (71 vs 71.7); higher body mass index (27.6 vs 26.5); and a prior fall within 12 months. Peripheral bone mass was not found to be a risk factor. Other large epidemiologic studies have demonstrated similar findings and many have theorized that obese elderly individuals at high risk for falls are at greater risk for ankle fractures than those with osteoporosis.[5,6] A comprehensive list of factors associated with elderly ankle fracture is shown in **Box 1**. In a more recent study, Pritchard and colleagues[7] followed a cohort of more than 3000 women older than age 50 for 5 years to assess the relationship between prior ankle fractures and a major osteoporotic fracture event (ie, hip or vertebral fractures). Ankle fractures did not predict future fragility fractures, but were associated with obesity and a history of prior

Funding Sources: Nil.
Conflicts of Interest: Nil.
[a] Department of Orthopaedics and Rehabilitation, University of Rochester Medical Center, 601 Elmwood Avenue, Rochester, NY 14642, USA; [b] American Orthopaedic Foot and Ankle Society, 6300 North River Road, Suite 510, Rosemont, IL 60018, USA
* Corresponding author.
E-mail address: Joshua_Olsen@urmc.rochester.edu

Orthop Clin N Am 44 (2013) 225–241
http://dx.doi.org/10.1016/j.ocl.2013.01.010
0030-5898/13/$ – see front matter Published by Elsevier Inc.

orthopedic.theclinics.com

Box 1
Patient factors associated with ankle fractures in the elderly

Risk Factors

- Smoking[8]
- Obesity[5–10]
- Vigorous physical activities[6]
- Sedentary individuals[6]
- Polypharmacy[8]
- Diabetes[10,11]
- Previous falls[5,6]
- Fracture history[7,8]
- Low bone mineral density at distal radius[6]
- Younger age[5]
- Female gender[10]

Protective Factors

- Vitamin D supplementation[6]
- Estrogen supplementation[6]
- Decreased weight gain[12]

fractures. Indeed, ankle fractures in the elderly are associated with risk factors that are different from osteoporotic hip and vertebral fractures.

Although osteoporosis is not a risk factor for ankle fractures, it is a risk factor for the failure of surgical fixation in ankle fractures. Difficulties with the fixation of osteoporotic ankle fractures are best highlighted by the varying opinions and surgical techniques in the orthopedic literature. Although some outcome studies suggest nonoperative management because of high surgical complications rates and failure of fixation, others suggest improved radiographic and clinical outcomes with surgical fixation. Opinions on the subject even vary with geographic location of the authors. Physicians on the west coast are more apt to surgically treat ankle fractures, whereas physicians on the east coast or with nearby teaching institutions are less apt to operate.[1] Surgical techniques range from standard plating with various methods of augmentation to locked plating technology to intramedullary nails to ankle fusions.

This article reviews the unique features of treating osteoporotic ankle fractures. It explores how to choose the best treatment plan based on the initial evaluation of the patient and anticipated outcomes. The difficulties of maintaining surgical fixation in osteoporotic ankle fracture are discussed and ways to augment fixation are shared. Finally, postoperative issues, such as time considerations for protected weight bearing and rehabilitation, are considered.

INITIAL EVALUATION

Elderly patients, with or without ankle fractures, tend to be osteoporotic. These patients' circumstances are complicated by several factors that must be identified in the initial assessment by the surgeon to develop a good treatment plan. Patient factors that must be identified include preinjury functional limitations, systemic medical problems, risk factors for fragility fractures, polypharmacy, cognitive changes, and end-of-life issues.[13] Obtaining an accurate history is a time-consuming process that always requires a thorough review of medical records and often requires the assistance of family members, healthcare proxies, and healthcare aides. In patients with dementia and a poor support network, the physician may have to rely solely on medical records, which may be incomplete. Medical consultation with an internist or geriatrician is an invaluable tool in the assessment process and is essential for managing the various medical issues unique to the elderly. At our institution, a protocol that involves early medical consultation within the emergency department for patients with geriatric hip fractures has proved to be effective and serves as a model for the management of trauma in the elderly.[14] Consultation with geriatricians in the management of nonhip fragility fractures is not automatically obtained at our institution, and there is currently no literature to suggest its effectiveness. Nonetheless, the success of our geriatric hip program has set the standard of care for geriatric trauma, and medical consultation is frequently sought in the management of elderly ankle fractures.

The second task when evaluating ankle fractures in the elderly is characterizing the injury itself. Some of these characteristics can be elucidated in the patient's history and include the mechanism and timing of injury, ability to ambulate after the injury, and history of osteoporosis. Other injury characteristics that the surgeon must know are determined by the physical examination. It is imperative to inspect the ankle for the quality of the soft tissue envelope and the presence of ulcers, blisters, or an open fracture. Light palpation of the foot, leg, and knee are important, as is a complete neurovascular examination. Testing with a 5.07 (10 g) Semmes Weinstein monofilament should be considered in patients suspected of peripheral neuropathy, and is imperative in all patients with diabetes. Peripheral vascular disease is not uncommon in the elderly and noninvasive vascular studies should be obtained in patients with diminished or absent pedal pulses, and in patients with ulcers or skin changes concerning for peripheral arterial disease. Vascular surgery consultation is recommended in patients with abnormal noninvasive vascular studies at our institution. The last component to a good examination is assessing the patient from head to toe to identify other associated injuries. Special attention should be paid to the head, proximal humerus, distal radius, and hip because these are frequently injured during ground level falls.[15]

Standard imaging should be obtained in all patients with ankle trauma and includes anteroposterior, mortise, and lateral views of the ankle, and radiographs of the foot and tibia. Advanced imaging, such as a computed tomography scan, is rarely needed, but may be helpful in assessing the size of a posterior malleolus fragment or assessing the joint if there is suspicion for intraarticular involvement. Stress or weight-bearing views can help distinguish between stable and unstable ankle injuries and can further guide treatment decisions.[16,17]

Most ankle fractures sustained in the elderly are lateral malleolus fractures.[18] There seems, however, to be a higher rate of complex ankle fractures in elderly patients compared with younger patients. In a retrospective comparison of patients that underwent surgical fixation of unstable ankle fractures, a higher occurrence of bimalleolar and trimalleolar fractures was observed in patients older than age 65 years versus patients younger than age 65 years.[19]

Any elderly patient being considered for surgery requires preoperative laboratory tests including a hematocrit, basic blood chemistries, and coagulation studies. In addition to these routine assessments, hemoglobin A_{1c} levels must be checked in all patients with diabetes to evaluate their overall glycemic control and predict their capacity to heal wounds.[20] Nutritional laboratory studies, such as serum albumin or total lymphocyte count, have been correlated with wound healing and may be helpful in patients with diabetes or who are malnourished.[21]

All elderly patients that sustain an ankle fracture require an evaluation of their overall bone health. Patients should be screened for a history of fragility fractures, prior bone mineral density scans, and prior use of medications for osteoporosis. Metabolic bone laboratory studies are recommended and include serum calcium, 25-hydroxyvitamin D, parathyroid hormone, and thyroid-stimulating hormone levels. Patients should be counseled about safe exercise and calcium and vitamin D supplementation, and encouraged to participate in fall-

reduction programs. It is imperative for orthopedic surgeons to play an active role in the diagnosis and education of osteoporosis, and refer untreated or undertreated patients at high risk for fragility fractures to their primary care physicians or metabolic bone clinics for appropriate treatment. The patient's past medical history, presentation, current medications, and past response to surgery, such as a prior nonunion, can prompt the treating orthopedist to obtain a more detailed medical work-up for osteoporosis.[22] Several programs, such as "Own the Bone," have been developed to help orthopedists identify and manage patients at high risk for future fragility fractures. Dell and colleagues[23] provide an excellent summary of osteoporosis, and spell out realistic goals for all orthopedists to accomplish in their practice. **Fig. 1** is a simple flowchart demonstrating how we typically evaluate patients suspected to have osteoporosis.

After the circumstances of the patient and characteristics of the injury have been fully assessed, the physician and patient (or patient's family) must make an informed decision between nonoperative or operative treatment plans. A dialogue with the patient and often the patient's family is beneficial and necessary to fully elicit a patient's wishes and address and answer all potential concerns or questions. The role of involving the patient's family or healthcare proxies becomes particularly more relevant in patients with cognitive dysfunction, codependence on family members for activities of daily living, or patients dealing with end-of-life issues. This is often a complex process, and should be guided by the surgeon's experience and knowledge of literature regarding outcomes in ankle fractures of the elderly.

OUTCOMES

In the past, many viewed operative fixation of ankle fractures in the elderly as imprudent secondary to the high rate of complications and marginal clinical outcomes reported in the literature. Beauchamp and colleagues[24] and Litchfield[25] retrospectively reviewed patients older than age 50 and 65 years, respectively, with unstable ankle fractures. Both studies reported high rates of deep infection (>11%) and malunion (>14%) in the operative group. Litchfield[25] reported only 58% of patients to have satisfactory results with surgery, and emphasized that patients with osteoporotic bone were likely to have poor clinical results. Beauchamp and colleagues[24] further questioned the role of surgery for ankle fractures in the elderly because the clinical outcomes between the operative and nonoperative groups were similar at

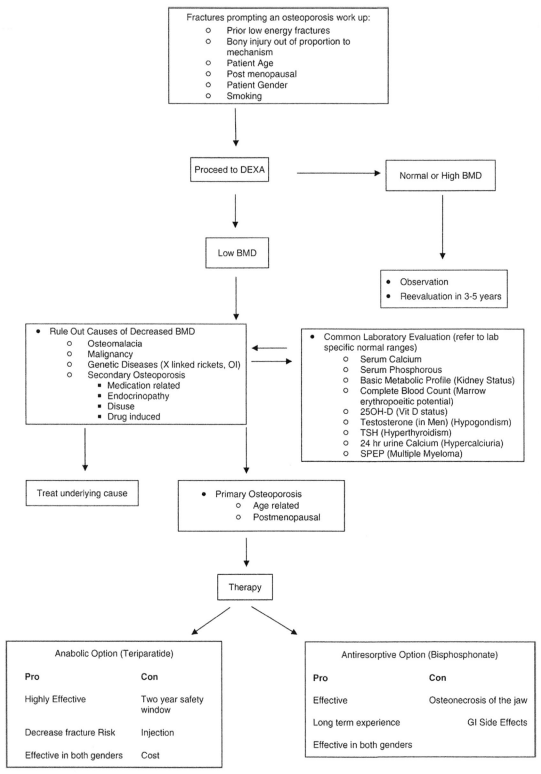

Fig. 1. A flowchart demonstrating how the authors typically evaluate patients suspected to have osteoporosis. BMD, bone mineral density; DEXA, dual-energy X-ray absorptiometry; GI, gastrointestinal; OI, osteogenesis imperfecta; SPEP, serum protein electrophoresis; TSH, thyroid-stimulating hormone. (*From* Patel A, Puzas E, Baumhauer J. Practical osteoporosis management: topical review. Foot Ankle Int 2010;31(4):354–60; with permission.)

2 years. Both studies failed to report on systemic illnesses; lacked validated outcome measures; and have been criticized for early, unprotected weight bearing as soon as 4 weeks following the operative procedure.

In a more recent prospective study by Salai and colleagues,[26] patients older than age 65 years with trimalleolar ankle fractures were randomized to treatment by either cast immobilization or internal fixation followed by cast immobilization for 6 weeks after initial stable reduction was achieved in the operating room by a senior orthopedic resident. At an average follow-up time of 37 months, the nonoperative group had a significantly better American Orthopedic Foot and Ankle Society score than the surgically treated group. Approximately 32% patients within the operative group required additional surgery for the removal of symptomatic hardware. The authors conclude that nonoperative treatment can provide superior clinical outcomes than surgery. This study failed to address systemic illnesses and 61% of patients within the operative group (30 of 49 patients) were surgically treated because of the inability to achieve an acceptable initial stable reduction in the operating room, thus leaving only 16 patients in the nonoperative group. Theoretically, the patients in the nonoperative group represented a more inherently stable fracture pattern than those patients treated surgically, and could represent a potential confounder in their final analysis between the groups.

The high complication rates and poor clinical outcomes associated with ankle fractures in an elderly population with osteoporosis are likely overstated in these studies. All three studies failed to account for the influence of systemic illnesses on complications rates; and all three studies used nonvalidated patient outcome measures. Moreover, the preponderance of literature suggests lower complication rates and better clinical outcomes than what is stated in these studies.

In a review of more than 33,000 patients from the Medicare national registry from 1998 to 2001 with an ankle fracture between the ages of 65 and 99 years, Koval and colleagues[18] reported an overall complication rate of 2% at 2 years in the operative group. The most common complication was hardware irritation (11%), and the most common reoperation was for removal of hardware (11%) over the course of 2 years. Rates of revision of internal fixation or other salvage procedures were less than 1%. Peripheral vascular disease, diabetes, and a Charlson index of one or more were predictive of a higher complication rate at 1 month and 1 year. Increasing age (per decade), peripheral vascular disease, diabetes, and a Charlson index

of one or more were predictive of higher mortality rates at 1 year. The overall mortality rates in the nonoperative and operative groups at 1 and 2 years were 9.2% and 16.1% versus 6.7% and 11.3%, respectively. The nonoperative group had a lower overall complication rate of 0.3%, but a higher overall mortality rate compared with the operative group. On average, the nonoperative group was older and had more medical comorbidities including diabetes and peripheral vascular disease.

Most publications on geriatric ankle fractures report favorable outcomes with surgery (**Table 1**).[19,27–35] Makwana and colleagues[28] randomly enrolled 43 patients older than age 55 with displaced ankle fractures after successful reduction into operative and nonoperative treatment groups. The surgical group was treated with a variety of techniques (semitubular plates, rush pins, kirschner wires) and immobilized for 2 weeks in a cast and then transitioned to full weight bearing under the supervision of a physiotherapist. The nonsurgical group was placed in a cast and made non–weight bearing for 6 weeks. Of the 21 patients initially treated with cast immobilization, eight patients required operative fixation for fracture displacement within 3 weeks. The patients within the operative group had better Olerud-Molander Ankle Scores (OMAS) and better ankle range of motion at 2 years of follow-up compared with the nonoperative group. Five patients were noted to have poor bone quality intraoperatively, but stable fixation and good outcomes were achieved in every case.

Advanced age does not seem to preclude good clinical outcomes with surgical fixation of ankle fractures. Shivarathre and colleagues[34] reviewed 82 patients older than age 80 years that underwent surgical fixation for unstable ankle fractures. Most patients (86%) returned to their preinjury mobility status. There was a low overall complication rate and superficial infection was the most common complication (7%). Four patients developed deep infection requiring hardware removal. Diabetes, peripheral vascular disease, dementia, and smoking were significantly associated with superficial and deep infections. Fong and colleagues[33] reported similar results in a small series of patients older than age 80 with unstable ankle fractures. Two of the 17 patients had deep infections and two patients had hardware failure. Of these four patients, three of the complications were attributed to osteopenia and premature weight bearing after surgery. The authors concluded that dementia and the patient's ability to follow instructions should be considered when choosing the appropriate treatment of ankle fractures in the

Table 1
A comprehensive list of outcome studies to date of ankle fracture in the elderly

Authors	LOE[66]	Population	Outcomes	Follow-up	Results	Recommend Surgery
Beauchamp et al,[24] 1983	Retrospective Level III	126 patients older than age 50	Clinical examination Complications Radiographs	~2 y	High rate of complications (61%), especially in women. 11.3% and 14.1% deep infection and malunion rates, respectively. *Allowed early unprotected weight bearing.*	No, especially in women
Litchfield,[25] 1987	Retrospective Level IV	31 patients older than age 65	Complications Radiographs	—	58% and 19% of patients had satisfactory and poor outcomes, respectively. 12.9% and 16.1% deep infection and malunion complication rates, respectively. *Allowed early unprotected weight bearing.*	No
Ali et al,[27] 1987	Retrospective Level III	100 patients older than age 60	Pain Stability Complications Radiographs	~7 y	Operative group had better pain control, clinical stability, and fewer malunions. 6% and 8.7% infection and malunion rate in operative group, respectively.	Yes
Salai et al,[26] 2000	Prospective Level II	84 patients older than age 65	AOFAS	~37 mo	AOFAS scores for the surgical group were 75 vs 91 for the nonsurgical group. 32% of surgical group required hardware removal for skin irritation over 2 y.	No
Makwana et al,[28] 2001	Prospective Level I	43 patients older than age 55	Clinical examination Radiographs OMAS VAS	~27 mo	8 of the 21 patients in the nonoperative group required surgery for fracture displacement in the first 3 weeks. 3 of 22 patients in the operative group underwent removal of symptomatic hardware. OMAS and ankle range of motion were significantly better in the operative group. Low complication rate in operative group.	Yes

Srinivasan & Moran,[29] 2001	Retrospective Level IV	74 patients older than age 70	Complications Length of stay Mobility Residential status Radiographs	—	85% of patients returned to preinjury mobility and residential status. Preinjury walker-use and open fractures were associated with longer hospital stays. Wound edge necrosis/delayed healing were seen in 9% of cases. Malunion rate of 5%. Deep infection rate of 1%. Osteoporotic bone precluded planned fixation in 12% and were treated in casts for 6–8 wk.	Yes
Pagliaro et al,[30] 2001	Retrospective Level IV	23 patients older than age 65	Complications Radiographs	~10 mo	One delayed union and wound dehiscence; two amputations; 8% deep infection rate and 4% SSI (one SSI). All complications associated with open injury, PVD, and diabetes. 0% malunion rate.	Yes
Vioreanu et al,[32] 2007	Retrospective Level III	112 patients older than age 70: 72 surgically and 40 with MUA and casting	Complications Mobility Additional procedures	16–22 wk	Operative treatment was associated with a higher return to preinjury mobility. Wound complications was the most common complication and one patient required a below-knee amputation. Nonoperative treatment was associated with a higher rate of additional surgery and a lower return to preinjury mobility.	Yes

(continued on next page)

Table 1
(continued)

Authors	LOE[66]	Population	Outcomes	Follow-up	Results	Recommend Surgery
Koval et al,[18] 2007	Retrospective Level III	33,704 patients from Medicare national registry between the ages of 65 and 99	Mortality Complications months after injury Additional surgery	6 mo–2 y	Patients treated operatively had higher rehospitalization rates at all time points. The overall complication rate was 2% at 2 y in the operative group vs 0.3% in the nonoperative group. Revision ankle surgery (internal fixation revision, arthrodesis, amputation) occurred in less than 1% of patients. 11% patients required hardware removal for irritation. Risk factors for increased mortality at 1 y included increasing age, diabetes, and PVD.	Low overall complication rates in the nonoperative and operative groups
Fong et al,[33] 2007	Retrospective Level IV	17 patients older than age 80	Complications Radiographs AOFAS	~18.5 mo	Four of the 17 patients had major complications requiring surgery: Two deep infections and two hardware failures. Three of the four complications were caused by patient noncompliance.	Yes
Anderson et al,[19] 2008	Retrospective Level III	25 patients older than age 65 and 46 patients ≤65 y of age	Complications Radiographs OMAS SF-36	~24–27 mo	Patients older than age 65 had more medical comorbidities, postoperative complications (40%), and higher need for nursing home placement (64%). Wound complications were the most common postoperative complication (20%). Long-term follow-up showed no difference in patient reported outcomes.	Yes

Study	Design/Level	Patients	Outcomes	Follow-up	Results	
Davidovitch et al,[31] 2009	Retrospective Level III	313 patients <60 vs 56 patients ≥60	Radiographs Complications AOFAS SMFA	12 mo	At 3 months, 57% of patients ≥60 y of reported activity limitations vs 33% of the patients younger than 60. Both groups returned to preinjury functional status. AOFAS scores were not significantly different at 3, 6, or 12 mo. 99% union rate overall at 1 y. 7% vs 13% overall complication rate not statistically different.	Yes
Shivarathre et al,[34] 2011	Retrospective Level IV	82 patients older than age 80	Mobility Complications Radiographs	~15 mo	7% superficial skin infections and 4% of patients developed deep infections requiring hardware removal. Diabetes, dementia, PVD, and smoking were significantly associated with superficial infections. 86% of patients returned to preinjury mobility status at 3–6 mo.	Yes
Lynde et al,[35] 2012	Retrospective Level IV	216 patients older than age 60	Complications	Minimum of 6 mo	The presence of comorbidities, early weight bearing, or locking vs nonlocking constructs was not correlated with a higher rate of postoperative complications. Complications were more common in older patients (73 vs 69 y of age). Wound dehiscence was the most common complication (10%) and diabetes was the only significant predictor for this complication.	Yes

Abbreviations: AOFAS, American Orthopedic Foot and Ankle Society; OMAS, Olerud-Molander Ankle Scores; PVD, peripheral vascular disease; SSI, surgical site infection.

elderly. Seven of the 17 patients were noted to have poor bone quality and were treated with various methods of augmented fixation including multiple syndesmotic screws, intramedullary fibular kirschner wires, and tension band wiring.

At the same institution that Beauchamp and colleagues[24] had previously reported on ankle fractures in the elderly in 1983, Srinivasan and Moran[29] reviewed 74 patients older than age 70 from 1989 to 1999 who underwent surgical fixation for unstable ankle fractures. Thirty-eight patients (51%) were initially treated with closed reduction and immobilization and subsequently required surgery for loss of reduction. Surgical fixation was abandoned in nine patients for poor bone quality and significant comminution and they were treated in a splint for 6 to 8 weeks. There was one case of deep infection (1%); four cases of malunion (5%); and seven cases of wound edge necrosis (9%). Most patients (85%) returned to their preinjury mobility and residential status. Hospital length of stay was significantly greater for patients requiring walkers before injury (112 days) than those who ambulated independently or with canes (19 days). The authors concluded that surgical fixation followed by 6 to 8 weeks of immobilization provides reasonable outcomes and low complications in the elderly.

Good results can be obtained with surgical fixation in elderly patients with unstable ankle fractures. Most patients report good outcomes, and return to their preinjury mobility and residential status. The overall complication rate is low in the elderly; hardware irritation, superficial infection, and skin edge necrosis are the most common complications. Higher rates of complications should be anticipated in patients with diabetes, dementia, peripheral vascular disease, and a history of smoking. In contrast to younger patients, elderly patients may require a longer hospital stay after surgery, and a longer period of postoperative immobilization compared with younger patients with similar injuries. The literature (see **Table 1**) seems to suggest that elderly patients have fewer complications and better outcomes if they are immobilized for 6 weeks or more. This period of immobilization is extended to 12 weeks at our institution after fixation of osteoporotic ankle fractures. This differs considerably from nonelderly patients because it is believed by many surgeons that early range of motion and weight bearing improves postoperative outcomes.[36]

There is no study to date that has specifically addressed the issue of poor bone quality and its effect on patient outcomes and complication rates. Osteopenia and osteoporosis pose a challenge to the surgeon to achieve stable fixation, but if stable fixation is achieved, these patients likely experience results similar to those without poor bone quality.

NONOPERATIVE MANAGEMENT

Stable ankle fractures should be treated nonoperatively and immobilized in a weight-bearing fiberglass cast. We prefer fiberglass casts to walking boots because they have a lower heel profile and reduce the risk of gait imbalance and subsequent falls. Nonoperative management for unstable ankle fractures should be strongly considered in patients confined to bed or wheelchair, and those that cannot undergo a surgical procedure safely secondary to health problems. Nonoperative management may also be considered in elderly patients with dementia who may not be able to follow postoperative instructions and rehabilitation protocols. Elderly patients with a myriad of comorbidities, such as diabetes mellitus, peripheral vascular disease, dementia, and tobacco dependence, should be offered surgery, but counseled about the higher risk of postoperative complications before obtaining informed consent. Superficial skin infection and hardware irritation are still the most common complications in this group; however, there seems to be a higher rate of deep infections, wound dehiscence, hardware failure, and amputations. Osteopenia or osteoporosis, by itself, is not a contraindication to surgical management of unstable ankle fractures.

OPERATIVE MANAGEMENT

Successful management of osteoporotic ankle fractures begins with good preoperative planning and adherence to basic fracture surgery principles. Nonetheless, achieving adequate fixation in osteoporotic bone can pose significant challenges despite advances in treatment strategies. Several surgical techniques have been developed to address this issue and provide the surgeon with a more effective armamentarium when treating these injuries. When adopting a new technique, it is important for the surgeon to consider their experience and comfort level with that technique, equipment availability, and implant costs.

FIXATION TECHNIQUES
Plate Osteosynthesis

The development of locking plate osteosynthesis has significantly improved fracture care in patients with osteoporosis. Conventional plating techniques rely on good frictional fit between the bone-plate interface to obtain adequate fixation. Frictional fit is highly dependent on bone mineral density. In comparison, locking plate technology creates a fixed angle construct and is not as dependent on bone mineral density to obtain adequate fixation.

Biomechanical studies have demonstrated the advantages of locking plates in osteoporotic distal fibula fractures. Zahn and colleagues[37] demonstrated in a cadaver model that contoured locking plates better resists external rotation forces in an axially loaded foot than conventional plating. Kim and colleagues[38] demonstrated that two unicortical locking screws placed in the distal fragment of the fibula are equivalent to three unicortical cancellous screws with respects to stiffness, load to failure, and torsional strength.

Plate position on the distal fibula can also improve stability. The antiglide technique has been shown to be superior in stiffness and load to failure for oblique distal fibula fractures than a lateral locking plate in osteoporotic bone.[39] These plates are placed posteriorly to accommodate fracture geometry, and allow ample soft tissue coverage of the plate, but may lead to peroneal tendon irritation. Minihane and colleagues[39] recommend using an antiglide plating technique if inadequate fixation of the distal fragment is achieved with locked lateral plating in patients with osteoporosis.

Despite their biomechanical advantages, a recent study by Schepers and colleagues[40] highlights an increased rate of wound complications when using locking plates. Two (1.2%) out of 165 patients in the one-third tubular group had deep infections necessitating hardware removal compared with 4 (10%) out of 40 in the locked plating group. One theory is that the overall thickness of locking plates can be twice that of conventional one-third tubular plates and lead to soft tissue irritation and possible skin breakdown. Although this study is underpowered, surgeons should pay close attention to plate thickness and its relationship to the overall size of the soft tissue envelope.

Tension-Band Technique

Several authors have investigated tension-band technique in the setting of ankle fractures in the elderly. Ostrum and Litsky[41] prospectively demonstrated good results in a study of 30 patients with a displaced medial malleolar fracture. Fracture union was achieved in all patients, and complications included one malunion and wound complication resulting in osteomyelitis. Georgiadis and White[42] reported "acceptable" outcomes with their tension band technique in a retrospective review of 22 patients. All fractures healed, and

complications included medial ankle pain related to prominent hardware, and asymptomatic wire migration. Johnson and Fallat[43] performed a biomechanical study comparing two cancellous screws with a tension band wiring technique to fix a displaced medial malleolus fracture. The tension band technique was four times as strong as the screws in a load to failure. All of these publications suggest that tension banding is useful for medial malleolar avulsion fractures; osteotomies; small transverse fracture fragments (in which a screw may cause iatrogenic fracture); or fixation of osteoporotic bone.[41–43]

Fibular Intramedullary Devices

Elderly patients tend to have frail skin and may be at increased risk for wound complications. One way to minimize the incision over the traumatized skin is to use intramedullary devices. The incision is small and typically distal to the site of traumatized skin.

Ramasamy and Sherry[44] treated nine patients with a 4.5-mm fibular nail and two distal locking screws, and allowed immediate weight bearing. They reported good to excellent results in 88% of patients (eight of nine) and improved OMAS. They cited the following advantages of fibular nailing in elderly patients: it provides (1) stable fixation of the lateral column; (2) better fixation in osteoporotic bones; (3) minimal soft tissue dissection and infection rate; and (4) and good to excellent results. These results were also seen in a group of 24 patients reported by Rajeev and colleagues.[45] They used a Biomet fibular nail and a single distal locking screw (± proximal blocking screw) and experienced no wound complications or nonunions at 1-year follow-up.

One potential complication of fibular nails is proximal migration of the nail with subsequent fibular shortening and talar tilt; this may be particularly true of unlocked nails. Bugler and colleagues[46] describe an evolution of their fibular nail locking technique in a review of 105 patients. A nonlocked fibular nail provided unsatisfactory results in four out of six patients (two patients with significant fixation failures) and so a variety of locking patterns were used. Techniques included a single distal locking screw, a distal locking screw with a proximal blocking screw, a single syndesmotic locking screw, and finally a distal locking screw in combination with a syndesmotic screw. They reported favorable OMAS with this technique and no skin complications. It is unclear as to the number or configuration of locking screws required to create a rotationally stable fibular nail, but it seems prudent to lock the nail above and below the fracture to maintain length and rotation of the fracture.

Arthrodesis

In general, arthrodesis is reserved for elderly patients with limited preinjury mobility and high mortality rates. Arthrodesis should almost never be considered in active and otherwise healthy elderly individuals with unstable ankle fractures.

Lemon and colleagues[47] performed ankle and subtalar fusions with an expandable calcaneotalotibial nail in 12 patients older than age 75 with unstable osteoporotic ankle fractures and allowed full weight bearing the day after surgery. Patients were recommended to have their nails removed at 12 weeks to avoid potential periprosthetic fractures, but six patients refused additional procedures. Results were overall favorable in terms of fusion success and OMAS at 67 weeks, and no complications were reported in 11 of 12 patients. One patient died 24 days after surgery from a myocardial infarction.

Amirfeyz and colleagues[48] reported similar results in their retrospective study of 13 patients. All patients available for final follow-up achieved radiographic union of their fusion sites and most returned to the preinjury functional status. One patient underwent revision nailing for valgus alignment; five patients died from unrelated causes. Postoperatively, patients remained partial weight bearing for 6 weeks and then were progressed to full weight bearing. Jonas and colleagues[49] retrospectively reviewed 31 patients with osteoporotic ankle fractures treated with calcaneotalotibial nails. There were three periprosthetic fractures, two broken nails, and two patients with symptomatic distal locking screws. Of the 21 patients with radiographic follow-up at approximately 8 months, 13 had radiographic union and 8 had no evidence of healing. Nonetheless, all patients returned to a functional level comparable with their preinjury status. Ten of the patients were too ill or deceased for follow-up. Given the issues with the implant and the high mortality rate, the authors recommend this technique in a patient demographic similar to those with geriatric hip fractures because it allows early weight bearing and there are few wound complications.

Ankle arthrodesis can also be used as a salvage technique in osteoporotic ankle fractures that failed primary fixation. Houshian and colleagues[50] report on four ill patients with osteoporotic bimalleolar ankle fractures that underwent initial fixation with a rush pin in the fibula and two kirschner wires in the medial malleolus. Postoperative films revealed fracture displacement and patients were elected to undergo arthrodesis with a calcaneotalotibial nail. Each patient had solid ankle fusions at 3 months, and all patients reported pain-free weight bearing at 12 months.

Steinmann Pin

Several authors have described a salvage procedure in which a vertical transtalar Steinmann pin is drilled in a retrograde manner through the calcaneus and into the tibia for stabilization of unstable ankle fractures.[51–53] This technique is reserved for elderly patients deemed inappropriate for internal fixation of their ankle fracture because of frail skin, severe soft tissue injury, and peripheral vascular disease. It also may serve a role in the polytrauma patient in which damage control orthopedic principles must be applied. Sciocsia and Ziran[53] used Steinmann pin fixation to further supplement their internal fixation in elderly patients with osteoporosis in the setting of pre-existing ankle osteoarthritis. This technique can serve a provisional or definitive role in the treatment of unstable ankle fractures and is typically removed at 6 weeks and patients are transitioned into a weight bearing boot or cast. Good overall results have been reported with this technique.[51]

External Fixators

External fixators are ideal in open ankle fractures. They allow convenient access to the soft tissues for appropriate monitoring and care. They also provide a good option of fixation in settings where the soft tissue envelope cannot accommodate a surgical incision. Surgical incisions should never be performed in ankle fractures with significant soft tissue swelling or bruising. Moreover, frail skin that is commonly encountered in the elderly may also be a relative contraindication to surgical incisions.

There is limited evidence in the literature regarding the use of hybrid or ringed fixators to primarily treat osteoporotic ankle fractures. The main theoretical advantage is multiple points of fixation without a surgical incision. Disadvantages include the overall size and weight of the construct and its deleterious effect on mobility, need for routine pin care, and pin-site infections.

AUGMENTATION TECHNIQUES
Bone Cements

Polymethyl methacrylate (PMMA), or conventional bone cement, is a nonabsorbable cement that greatly increases the holding power of screw fixation in osteoporotic bone.[54] It has a good track record in several case series[55,56]; almost every orthopedist has some experience with handling characteristics of PMMA. Nonetheless, PMMA has its disadvantages. PMMA cures by an exothermic reaction, which may lead to thermal necrosis and subsequently impair bony healing.[57,58] It is nonabsorbable and can be a challenge to remove during revision surgery. Lastly, it can be difficult to achieve the proper consistency needed to sufficiently fill and augment screw holes.

Commercially available calcium phosphate cements (CPC) provide an attractive alternative to PMMA. They are bioresorbable, cure by an endothermic process, and are structurally similar to cancellous bone when hardened. CPC may have favorable handling characteristics to that of PMMA because it is delivered as an injectable paste and drillable after it hardens.[59] It demonstrates comparable screw pull out strength to that of PMMA, and has superior compressive strength to that of cancellous bone autograft.[54,60] Although promising, CPC is expensive and there are little clinical data to support its use in the treatment of osteoporotic ankle fractures.

Bone quality is the ultimate determine in screw pull out strength. Collinge and colleagues[54] performed a biomechanical study to assess screw pull out strength between tricalcium phosphate and PMMA in locked and nonlocked constructs. Locked plates augmented with either cement demonstrated improved biomechanical strength compared with conventional plating with or without cement. Nonetheless, the construct always failed at the bone-cement or bone-screw interface. It never failed at the cement-screw interface. This study highlights the concept of bone quality being the absolute determinant in screw purchase.

Screw Anchors

Some investigators have devised nylon cavity plugs, which are inserted into the medullary canal after predrilling of the cortex.[61] Early studies have shown promising results with improved resistance to screw pullout, but these products are early in their development, and currently not commercially available.

Permutations

The use of several augmentation techniques at once may be advantageous in the treatment of osteoporotic ankle fractures. This could include supplementing initial internal fixation with external fixators, bone cements, or intramedullary pins.

Assal and colleagues[62] retrospectively looked at displaced lateral malleolar fractures in the setting of osteoporosis. They showed good results using fixation consisting of a lateral plate and screws, which were augmented with PMMA, and a 2.5-mm terminally threaded intramedullary wire inserted retrograde into the fibula. They had 100% union rate (N = 36) at 6 months with full weight bearing at a mean of 13.5 days with 90% of patients returning to their preinjury ambulatory level.

Interpreting the clinical use of augmenting initial fixation with cement and pins from this study is difficult because the sample size is small and there are no control subjects. Additional research is needed in this area to validate the use of multiple augmentation techniques to supplement initial internal fixation in osteoporotic ankle fractures.

Our Preferred Technique

At our institution, osteoporotic ankle fractures are commonly treated with a technique we have coined the "comb technique." In this technique, multiple syndesmotic screws are used proximally, and locking screws are used in the distal fragment (Fig. 2). The number of syndesmotic screws is determined at the time of surgery and depends on bone quality and screw purchase. Our goal is to achieve maximal fixation in these patients, and we routinely fill every proximal screw hole with four-cortices syndesmotic screw if it provides better overall fixation.

The medial malleolar fracture can be fixed well with fully threaded cancellous screws through a well-reduced fragment. Despite the screw being fully threaded, we still get compression through the fracture fragment because of the poor bone quality, and this ensures good fixation to the distal tibia. The medial malleolar fragment may also be fixed with a bicortical screw, which has demonstrated favorable biomechanical properties to a partially threaded lag screw, or tension band techniques.[63]

In the setting of failed internal fixation, severe comminution, or marked osteoporosis our preferred method of salvage is primary fusion of the ankle and subtalar joints with a calcaneotalotibial nail (Fig. 3). One could argue not to violate the subtalar joint because it is not primarily involved with an ankle fracture. Patients who fail initial fixation because of extremely poor bone quality tend to be lower demand and sicker patients. Similar to elderly patients with hip fractures, early weight bearing is important to limit potential complications that occur from immobility. Fusing the subtalar and ankle joints with a load-sharing device, such as a nail, is a strong construct and allows early weight bearing and may be advantageous in this patient population. One of the major late complications from an ankle fusion is the development of subtalar arthritis. In this patient population

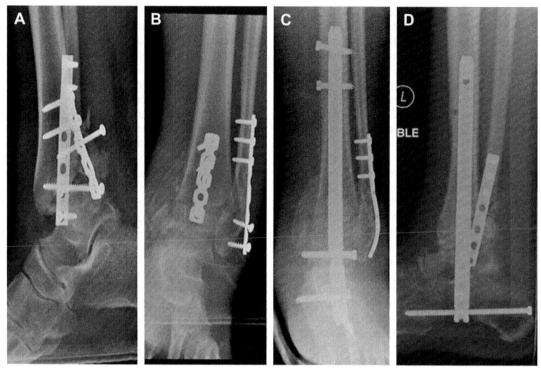

Fig. 2. A 45-year-old woman with diabetes mellitus, renal failure, and osteoporosis who suffered a posterior and lateral malleolar fracture that was repaired initially with open reduction and internal fixation (ORIF). (*A, B*) Four weeks postoperatively her fixation failed and she sustained a trimalleolar ankle. (*C, D*) She was revised with ankle and subtalar arthrodesis as a salvage technique and went on to uneventful union. (*Courtesy of* John Ketz, MD.)

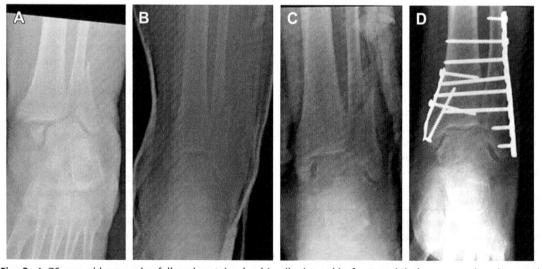

Fig. 3. A 76-year-old man who fell and sustained a bimalleolar ankle fracture (*A*) that was reduced treated initially in a short leg splint and strict non–weight bearing (*B*). Despite patient compliance, the reduction was lost 10 days later (*C*) and he was referred to our division for management. (*D*) He was treated with the "comb technique" using five syndesmotic screws and a 4.5 locking plate laterally and fully threaded cancellous screw medially, in addition to plate and screw fixation medially. Patient is currently 8 months postoperatively and doing well. (*Courtesy of* John Ketz, MD.)

with the metabolically weaker bone and the stress transfer from an ankle fusion, the subtalar joint is particularly vulnerable. No studies have been published on this issue to date in this patient population.

POSTOPERATIVE CARE

All unstable ankle malleolar fractures treated with internal fixation are kept non–weight bearing for 6 to 8 weeks in a plaster splint or fiberglass cast and then transitioned to a walking cast or boot for 4 weeks. Standard of care dictates that all patients receive perioperative antibiotics, deep venous thrombosis (DVT) prophylaxis, and calcium and vitamin D supplementation. All patients are seen by physical therapy on the day after surgery to assess their ambulatory status and identify rehabilitation needs. Medical comorbidities and postoperative issues (ie, hyponatremia, delirium, and urinary retention) should be comanaged with the hospitalist or geriatrician. Lastly, good communication with the patient, patient's family, or healthcare proxy is essential to the overall care of the patient and must not be overlooked.

Unlike our geriatric hip fracture program, we do not have a standardized protocol for DVT prophylaxis in patients with osteoporotic ankle fractures at our institution. Elderly patients with hip fractures routinely receive 6 weeks of low-molecular-weight heparin (LMWH). There is no consensus among surgeons regarding DVT prophylaxis in patients with immobilized lower extremities. Two meta-analyses recommend the use of LMWH because it decreases the rate of DVT and has a low bleeding complication rate.[64,65] Pooling data from heterogeneous patient populations to create recommendations and then applying it to specific patient populations are always problematic. Despite the limitations, we routinely use LMWH in poorly mobile elderly patients who are immobilized for their ankle fracture. We do not use LMWH in patients at risk for bleeding complications.

SUMMARY

Surgical treatment of unstable ankle fractures in osteoporotic patients can be challenging, but rewarding. Good outcomes and low overall complication rates can be achieved with good preoperative care and surgical planning. Good preoperative care includes identifying risk factors, such as diabetes, peripheral vascular disease, and dementia, and obtaining early medical consultation to help comanage these issues during the perioperative period. Identifying risk factors also helps surgeons educate patients and families

regarding outcomes and complications. Common complications include hardware irritation, superficial infections, and wound edge necrosis, and the less common complication of hardware failure and the need for future surgery. It is also essential for surgeons to take an active role in identifying and treating osteoporosis.

Several surgical techniques and implants have been developed to help surgeons achieve stable fixation in osteoporotic bone. It is important to anticipate the need for any special equipment (type of plate, nails, cements, and so forth) before the operating room to better accommodate decisions that are made at the time of surgery. Furthermore, if initial fixation fails, take heart; several salvage procedures for failed internal fixation have been described with reasonable outcomes.

REFERENCES

1. Koval KJ, Lurie J, Zhou W, et al. Ankle fractures in the elderly: what you get depends on where you live and who you see. J Orthop Trauma 2005;19: 635–9.
2. Kannus P, Palvanen M, Niemi S, et al. Increasing number and incidence of low-trauma ankle fractures in elderly people: Finnish statistics during 1970-2000 and projections for the future. Bone 2002;31: 430–3.
3. Kannus P, Palvanen M, Niemi S, et al. Stabilizing incidence of low-trauma ankle fractures in elderly people Finnish statistics in 1970-2006 and prediction for the future. Bone 2008;43:340–2.
4. Burge R, Dawson-Hughes B, Solomon DH, et al. Incidence and economic burden of osteoporosis-related fractures in the United States, 2005-2025. J Bone Miner Res 2007;22:465–75.
5. Hasselman CT, Vogt MT, Stone KL, et al. Foot and ankle fractures in elderly white women. Incidence and risk factors. J Bone Joint Surg Am 2003;85:820–4.
6. Seeley DG, Kelsey J, Jergas M, et al. Predictors of ankle and foot fractures in older women. The Study of Osteoporotic Fractures Research Group. J Bone Miner Res 1996;11:1347–55.
7. Pritchard JM, Giangregorio LM, Ioannidis G, et al. Ankle fractures do not predict osteoporotic fractures in women with or without diabetes. Osteoporos Int 2012;23:957–62.
8. Valtola A, Honkanen R, Kröger H, et al. Lifestyle and other factors predict ankle fractures in perimenopausal women: a population-based prospective cohort study. Bone 2002;30:238–42.
9. Greenfield DM, Eastell R. Risk factors for ankle fracture. Osteoporos Int 2001;12:97–103.
10. Daly PJ, Fitzgerald RH, Melton LJ, et al. Epidemiology of ankle fractures in Rochester, Minnesota. Acta Orthop Scand 1987;58:539–44.

11. Schwartz AV, Sellmeyer DE, Ensrud KE, et al. Older women with diabetes have an increased risk of fracture: a prospective study. J Clin Endocrinol Metab 2001;86:32–8.

12. Margolis KL, Ensrud KE, Schreiner PJ, et al. Body size and risk for clinical fractures in older women. Study of Osteoporotic Fractures Research Group. Ann Intern Med 2000;133:123–7.

13. Koval KJ, Meek R, Schemitsch E, et al. An AOA critical issue. Geriatric trauma: young ideas. J Bone Joint Surg Am 2003;85:1380–8.

14. Friedman SM, Mendelson DA, Kates SL, et al. Geriatric co-management of proximal femur fractures: total quality management and protocol-driven care result in better outcomes for a frail patient population. J Am Geriatr Soc 2008;56:1349–56.

15. Clement ND, Aitken S, Duckworth AD, et al. Multiple fractures in the elderly. J Bone Joint Surg Br 2012; 94:231–6.

16. Hoshino CM, Nomoto EK, Norheim EP, et al. Correlation of weightbearing radiographs and stability of stress positive ankle fractures. Foot Ankle Int 2012; 33:92–8.

17. van den Bekerom MP, Mutsaerts EL, van Dijk CN. Evaluation of the integrity of the deltoid ligament in supination external rotation ankle fractures: a systematic review of the literature. Arch Orthop Trauma Surg 2009;129:227–35.

18. Koval KJ, Zhou W, Sparks MJ, et al. Complications after ankle fracture in elderly patients. Foot Ankle Int 2007;28:1249–55.

19. Anderson SA, Li X, Franklin P, et al. Ankle fractures in the elderly: initial and long-term outcomes. Foot Ankle Int 2008;29:1184–8.

20. Christman AL, Selvin E, Margolis DJ, et al. Hemoglobin A1c predicts healing rate in diabetic wounds. J Invest Dermatol 2011;131:2121–7.

21. Koval KJ, Maurer SG, Su ET, et al. The effects of nutritional status on outcome after hip fracture. J Orthop Trauma 1999;13:164–9.

22. Tosi LL, Gliklich R, Kannan K, et al. The American Orthopaedic Association's "own the bone" initiative to prevent secondary fractures. J Bone Joint Surg Am 2008;90:163–73.

23. Dell RM, Greene D, Anderson D, et al. Osteoporosis disease management: What every orthopaedic surgeon should know? The Journal of Bone and Joint Surgery. American 2009;91(Suppl 6):79–86.

24. Beauchamp CG, Clay NR, Thexton PW. Displaced ankle fractures in patients over 50 years of age. J Bone Joint Surg Br 1983;65:329–32.

25. Litchfield JC. The treatment of unstable fractures of the ankle in the elderly. Injury 1987;18:128–32.

26. Salai M, Dudkiewicz I, Novikov I, et al. The epidemic of ankle fractures in the elderly: is surgical treatment warranted? Arch Orthop Trauma Surg 2000;120: 511–3.

27. Ali MS, McLaren CA, Rouholamin E, et al. Ankle fractures in the elderly: nonoperative or operative treatment. J Orthop Trauma 1987;1:275–80.

28. Makwana NK, Bhowal B, Harper WM, et al. Conservative versus operative treatment for displaced ankle fractures in patients over 55 years of age. A prospective, randomised study. J Bone Joint Surg Br 2001;83:525–9.

29. Srinivasan CM, Moran CG. Internal fixation of ankle fractures in the very elderly. Injury 2001;32:559–63.

30. Pagliaro AJ, Michelson JD, Mizel MS. Results of operative fixation of unstable ankle fractures in geriatric patients. Foot Ankle Int 2001;22:399–402.

31. Davidovitch RI, Walsh M, Spitzer A, et al. Functional outcome after operatively treated ankle fractures in the elderly. Foot Ankle Int 2009;30:728–33.

32. Vioreanu M, Brophy S, Dudeney S, et al. Displaced ankle fractures in the geriatric population: operative or non-operative treatment. Foot Ankle Surg 2007; 13:10–4.

33. Fong W, Acevedo JI, Stone RG, et al. The treatment of unstable ankle fractures in patients over eighty years of age. Foot Ankle Int 2007;28:1256–9.

34. Shivarathre DG, Chandran P, Platt SR. Operative fixation of unstable ankle fractures in patients aged over 80 years. Foot Ankle Int 2011;32:599–602.

35. Lynde MJ, Sautter T, Hamilton GA, et al. Complications after open reduction and internal fixation of ankle fractures in the elderly. Foot Ankle Surg 2012;18:103–7.

36. Lin CW, Donkers NA, Refshauge KM, et al. Rehabilitation for ankle fractures in adults. Cochrane Database Syst Rev 2012;(11):CD005595.

37. Zahn RK, Frey S, Jakubietz RG, et al. A contoured locking plate for distal fibular fractures in osteoporotic bone: a biomechanical cadaver study. Injury 2011;43:718–25.

38. Kim T, Ayturk UM, Haskell A, et al. Fixation of osteoporotic distal fibula fractures: a biomechanical comparison of locking versus conventional plates. J Foot Ankle Surg 2007;46:2–6.

39. Minihane KP, Lee C, Ahn C, et al. Comparison of lateral locking plate and antiglide plate for fixation of distal fibular fractures in osteoporotic bone: a biomechanical study. J Orthop Trauma 2006;20:562–6.

40. Schepers T, Van Lieshout EM, De Vries MR, et al. Increased rates of wound complications with locking plates in distal fibular fractures. Injury 2011;42:1125–9.

41. Ostrum RF, Litsky AS. Tension band fixation of medial malleolus fractures. J Orthop Trauma 1992; 6:464–8.

42. Georgiadis GM, White DB. Modified tension band wiring of medial malleolar ankle fractures. Foot Ankle Int 1995;16:64–8.

43. Johnson BA, Fallat LM. Comparison of tension band wire and cancellous bone screw fixation for medial malleolar fractures. J Foot Ankle Surg 1997;36:284–9.

44. Ramasamy PR, Sherry P. The role of a fibular nail in the management of Weber type B ankle fractures in elderly patients with osteoporotic bone: a preliminary report. Injury 2001;32:477–85.

45. Rajeev A, Senevirathna S, Radha S, et al. Functional outcomes after fibula locking nail for fragility fractures of the ankle. J Foot Ankle Surg 2011;50:547–50.

46. Bugler KE, Watson CD, Hardie AR, et al. The treatment of unstable fractures of the ankle using the Acumed fibular nail: development of a technique. J Bone Joint Surg Br 2012;94:1107–12.

47. Lemon M, Somayaji HS, Khaleel A, et al. Fragility fractures of the ankle: stabilisation with an expandable calcaneotalotibial nail. J Bone Joint Surg Br 2005;87:809–13.

48. Amirfeyz R, Bacon A, Ling J, et al. Fixation of ankle fragility fractures by tibiotalocalcaneal nail. Arch Orthop Trauma Surg 2008;128:423–8.

49. Jonas SC, Young AF, Curwen CH, et al. Functional outcome following tibio-talar-calcaneal nailing for unstable osteoporotic ankle fractures. Injury 2012. [Epub ahead of print].

50. Houshian S, Bajaj SK, Mohammed AM. Salvage of osteoporotic ankle fractures after failed primary fixation with an ankle arthrodesis nail: a report on four cases. Injury 2006;37:791–4.

51. Childress HM. Vertical transarticular pin fixation for unstable ankle fractures: impressions after 16 years of experience. Clin Orthop Relat Res 1976;164–71.

52. Morgan-Jones RL, Smith KD, Thomas PB. Vertical transtalar Steinmann pin fixation for unstable ankle fractures. Ann R Coll Surg Engl 2000;82:185–9.

53. Scioscia TN, Ziran BH. Use of a vertical transarticular pin for stabilization of severe ankle fractures. Am J Orthop (Belle Mead NJ) 2003;32:46–8.

54. Collinge C, Merk B, Lautenschlager EP. Mechanical evaluation of fracture fixation augmented with tricalcium phosphate bone cement in a porous osteoporotic cancellous bone model. J Orthop Trauma 2007; 21:124–8.

55. Schatzker J, Ha'eri GB, Chapman M. Methylmethacrylate as an adjunct in the internal fixation of intertrochanteric fractures of the femur. J Trauma 1978; 18:732–5.

56. Struhl S, Szporn MN, Cobelli NJ, et al. Cemented internal fixation for supracondylar femur fractures in osteoporotic patients. J Orthop Trauma 1990;4: 151–7.

57. Van Landuyt P, Peter B, Beluze L, et al. Reinforcement of osteosynthesis screws with brushite cement. Bone 1999;25:95S–8S.

58. Leeson MC, Lippitt SB. Thermal aspects of the use of polymethylmethacrylate in large metaphyseal defects in bone. A clinical review and laboratory study. Clin Orthop Relat Res 1993;239–45.

59. Larsson S, Procter P. Optimising implant anchorage (augmentation) during fixation of osteoporotic fractures: is there a role for bone-graft substitutes? Injury 2011;42(Suppl 2):S72–6.

60. Trenholm A, Landry S, McLaughlin K, et al. Comparative fixation of tibial plateau fractures using alpha-BSM, a calcium phosphate cement, versus cancellous bone graft. J Orthop Trauma 2005;19:698–702.

61. Drew T, Allcock P. A new method of fixation in osteoporotic bone. A preliminary report. Injury 2002;33: 685–9.

62. Assal M, Christofilopoulos P, Lübbeke A, et al. Augmented osteosynthesis of OTA 44-B fractures in older patients: a technique allowing early weight-bearing. J Orthop Trauma 2011;25:742–7.

63. Ricci WM, Tornetta P, Borrelli J. Lag screw fixation of medial malleolar fractures: a biomechanical, radiographic, and clinical comparison of unicortical partially threaded lag screws and bicortical fully threaded lag screws. J Orthop Trauma 2012;26: 602–6.

64. Ettema HB, Kollen BJ, Verheyen CC, et al. Prevention of venous thromboembolism in patients with immobilization of the lower extremities: a meta-analysis of randomized controlled trials. J Thromb Haemost 2008;6:1093–8.

65. Testroote M, Stigter W, de Visser DC, et al. Low molecular weight heparin for prevention of venous thromboembolism in patients with lower-leg immobilization. Cochrane Database Syst Rev 2008;(4):CD006681.

66. Wright JG, Swiontkowski MF, Heckman JD. Introducing levels of evidence to the journal. J Bone Joint Surg Am 2003;85:1–3.

Surgical Stabilization of the Spine in the Osteoporotic Patient

Shah-Nawaz M. Dodwad, MD, Safdar N. Khan, MD*

KEYWORDS

• Osteoporosis • Fracture • Surgical fixation • Fusion

KEY POINTS

- Ten million Americans have been diagnosed with osteoporosis, and an additional 34 million Americans are at risk for developing osteoporosis. The economic costs of osteoporosis-related fractures were $19 billion in 2005 and are predicted to increase to $25.3 billion by 2025.
- Osteoporosis places a patient at risk of fracture, progression of deformity, and difficulty with surgical fixation.
- Indications for surgical intervention in osteoporotic patients are similar to non-osteoporotic patients and include radiculopathy, myelopathy, mechanical back pain, progressive spinal deformity with or without fracture, neurogenic claudication, and failure of conservative management.
- Although the risks are higher in osteoporotic patients, once stable fixation and fusion has been achieved, patients' self-reported health assessments significantly improve with respect to physical function, social function, bodily pain, and perceived health change.
- Treating the osteoporotic spine patient involves a multidisciplinary approach with involvement of the primary care physician, endocrinologist, and physical therapist.

INTRODUCTION

Osteoporosis is the most common metabolic bone disorder. The National Osteoporosis Foundation defines osteoporosis as "porous bone ... a disease characterized by low bone mass and structural deterioration of bone tissue, leading to bone fragility and an increased susceptibility to fractures, especially of the hip, spine and wrist, although any bone can be affected."[1] The National Institutes of Health defines osteoporosis as the "thinning of bone tissue and loss of bone density over time."[2] Using the young adult mean bone mineral density (BMD) as a reference, the World Health Organization has defined osteoporosis more objectively as having a T score of less than −2.5. This score indicates a BMD less than 2.5 SDs below the BMD of an average 25-year-old adult.[3] According to the National Osteoporosis Foundation, 10 million Americans have been diagnosed with osteoporosis and an additional 34 million Americans are at risk for developing osteoporosis. The economic costs of osteoporosis-related fractures were $19 billion in 2005. These costs are predicted to increase to $25.3 billion by 2025. There were 2 million osteoporosis-related fractures in 2005, of which 547,000 were vertebral fractures.[1]

Similar to diabetes, osteoporosis is often a silent disease, frequently diagnosed after a clinically evident fracture occurs. Osteoporotic spine fractures can manifest as compression fractures, burst fractures, and sacral insufficiency fractures. Osteoporotic patients not only have bone disease, but, because of the skewed advanced age of this population, often have additional comorbid conditions that increase their overall operative risk. In addition to co-morbid conditions, core weakness

Department of Orthopaedics, The Ohio State University, Columbus, OH, USA
* Corresponding author. Department of Orthopaedics, The Ohio State University, 725 Prior Hall, 376 West Tenth Street, Columbus, OH 43210.
E-mail address: safdar.khan@osumc.edu

Orthop Clin N Am 44 (2013) 243–249
http://dx.doi.org/10.1016/j.ocl.2013.01.008
0030-5898/13/$ – see front matter © 2013 Elsevier Inc. All rights reserved.

in this patient population can lead to postoperative problems, hindering recovery and often necessitating inpatient rehabilitation.[4,5] Understandably, mortality after clinical vertebral fracture is increased.[6] Kado and colleagues[7] looked at 9575 women for more than 8 years and found that 1 vertebral column fracture increased mortality rates 23% to 34%. Given the prevalence, morbidity, and mortality involved with osteoporosis, screening and treatment are paramount.

Knowing the socioeconomic burden of osteoporotic fractures and deformity, spine surgeons must be trained and prepared to treat these patients. It is the aim of this article to remind and inform spine surgeons of osteoporosis and operative techniques that exist to help provide osteoporotic patients excellent and comprehensive care of their disease.

OSTEOPOROSIS

There are 3 types of osteoporosis. Type I, or postmenopausal, occurs in women or hypogonadic men. The primary hormonal imbalance is a decrease in estrogen. The fractures involved generally occur between 50 and 60 years of age, predominantly in the wrist and spine. Type II or senile osteoporosis occurs in men and women around 70+ years of age. Type III or secondary osteoporosis occurs because of other medical conditions or treatments, most commonly steroid-induced osteoporosis.[8]

The basic pathologic condition involves an imbalance between bone formation and resorption whereby the latter is in favor, resulting in a loss in bone mineral density over time. Although adults lose bone mass at 0.5% per year, not every individual develops osteoporosis. Rather, osteoporosis is multifactorial, involving environment, lifestyle, genetic, hormonal, medication, nutrition, and other disease processes.[9–12] The underlying concepts behind these pathophysiologic causes of osteoporosis are peak bone mass and rate of bone loss.[13] Not only does osteoporosis place a patient at risk of fracture, but also, once a fracture occurs, surgical fixation can be difficult. In addition, osteoporosis can cause progression of deformity by gradual loss of height within the spinal column.[14]

MEDICAL OPTIMIZATION

If possible, before surgical intervention, medical management of osteoporosis and other comorbidities must be optimized. These patients should be aware that they are at increased surgical risk because of their age.[15] Involvement of the primary care physician and an endocrinologist is key in this multidisciplinary approach to spinal care. Treatment begins with calcium and vitamin D

supplementation to decrease the rate of bone resorption and to mineralize osteoid. In select patients, hormone replacement therapy with selective estrogen receptor modulators can be beneficial.[16] Bisphosphonates, calcitonin, and parathyroid hormone therapies play key roles in osteoporosis treatment.[17–19]

Controversy exists with patients actively taking bisphosphonates as they may inhibit or delay spinal fusion. In 2005, Huang and colleagues[20] performed an animal study showing that alendronate, in a dose-dependent fashion, showed increased bone mass area but inhibited actual bone fusion in the spine by nearly 50% at 8 weeks. At the time, they recommended that patients should not take alendronate until bone fusion is achieved. Similarly, in 2004 Lehman and colleagues[21] used an animal study to show alendronate delayed or inhibited bone fusion in the spine. They thought this was the result of uncoupling of the osteoclastic and osteoblastic cells needed for bone healing and also recommended that alendronate should not be given in the acute fusion period.

However, in the osteoporotic spine, bisphosphonate therapy may actually be beneficial. In 2011, Nagahama and colleagues[22] showed that in a prospective randomized control study of 40 osteoporotic patients, 95% of the alendronate patients and 65% of the control patients had achieved bone fusion at 1 year. Although there was a trend toward better clinical outcomes in the alendronate group, there was no statistically significant difference in clinical outcomes. They concluded that osteoporotic patients should take bisphosphonates throughout the postoperative period. In addition, in 2011, Nakao and colleagues[23] assessed spinal fusion in osteoporotic rats and also concluded that alendronate may improve spine fusion healing in the presence of osteoporosis.

A discussion should occur with the endocrinologist as to whether they feel the bisphosphonate patient should switch to another anti-osteoporotic medication in the postoperative period. Future medical therapies on the horizon include antibodies directed against the endogenous inhibitors of bone formation.[24] In addition, physical therapy and Tai Chi improve patient strength, balance, and proprioception, which not only aid in fracture prevention but also help in postoperative rehabilitation.[25–27]

SURGICAL TECHNIQUES IN THE OSTEOPOROTIC SPINE

The indications for surgical intervention are similar to a nonosteoporotic patient population and include radiculopathy, myelopathy, mechanical back pain, progressive spinal deformity with or without fracture, neurogenic claudication, and failure of conservative management. A thorough risk-benefit analysis is required before operating on an osteoporotic patient. Although the risks are higher in this surgical population, once stable fixation and fusion have been achieved, patients' self-reported health assessments significantly improve with respect to physical function, social function, bodily pain, and perceived health change.[28] In the study by Okuda and colleagues,[29] fusion rates in patients older than 70 were delayed in 10%, had collapsed union in 13%, but had similar fusion rates to patients younger than 70 (100%). Surgical treatment of this patient population is a reasonable and viable option in the appropriately selected patient.[30]

Once conservative management has failed and appropriate time for medical optimization has been met, a spine surgeon must carefully plan their surgical intervention. Less is often more in deformity correction in the osteoporotic spine. Aggressive deformity correction can lead to implant overload and hardware failure. Major corrections should be avoided in favor of limited corrections. For example, when dealing with spinal stenosis, a greater attempt should be made to try to identify the specific level or nerve root of pathologic abnormality or the area of worst compression to have a 1-level or 2-level decompression, rather than large multilevel decompressions. Some surgeons may discuss in situ fusion when a significant concern exists of instrumentation failure because of abnormal bone or where the risk of progressive deformity is low.[31] The specific criteria for in situ fusion remain open for discussion. In 1992, Lenke and colleagues[32] looked at 56 isthmic spondylolisthesis patients and had an in situ fusion rate of about 50% but despite this low fusion rate they had improvement in clinical outcomes in greater than 80% of their patients. In situ fusion is simply 1 tool a spine surgeon can use when needed.

Another option for osteoporotic patients is to increase the extent of surgery by performing combined anterior/posterior intervention. A 360° fusion allows load-sharing and places less strain on the posterior-only fixation, yielding a more stable construct. Caution must be used with anterior interbody devices as they may subside in the weak osteoporotic bone. Given that the cortical bone is usually stronger in osteoporotic spine, anterior implants should have an appropriate size or footprint to engage this stronger cortical bone. The potential benefit of using anterior interbody load-sharing devices must be weighed against the increased risk to this medically fragile patient population from increased operative time, blood loss, and overall surgical risk. In addition, osteotomy may be used to correct deformity and decrease strain on the hardware.

The level at which to end the construct is critical in all spine patients. However, in the osteoporotic patient with poor bone mineral density and weaker bone it is even more important to take into account the junctional strain placed at the end levels of a construct. Increased strain at spinal transition zones should be avoided. Ending the cephalad portion of lumbar constructs at L1 should be avoided. Rather, T10 should be used to avoid kyphotic collapse at the thoracolumbar transition zone. The caudal aspect of cervical constructs should extend into T2 rather than ending at C7 to again avoid junctional kyphosis at the cervicothoracic transition point.

Given that insertional torque, pullout strength, and fatigue failure are linearly related to bone mineral density, the weakest link in fixation of the osteoporotic spine is the bone-implant interface.[33] The most common mechanism of bone-implant failure in the osteoporotic spine is screw pullout or cutout. Many techniques have been described to augment fixation, including cement augmentation with polymethylmethacrylate (PMMA) into pedicle screw tracks, hydroxyapatite-coated screws, sublaminar hooks and wiring, cross-linking, and expandable screws and screw design.

In most cases, better screw fixation is achieved with greater outer screw diameter. In addition, the tactile screw purchase achieved may be a reasonable indication of fixation. Screw placement with an insertional screw torque of less than 4 inch-pounds is likely to fail.[34] Some literature suggests that insertional screw torque may not be completely reliable to assess fixation as screw design may alter insertional torque such that certain screws may have higher insertional torques with a decreased pullout strength compared with other screws.[35]

Given the risk of bicortical purchase in pedicle screw placement, surgeons should aim for 80% vertebral body pedicle screw length. Medially angulated pedicle screws in a triangular configuration with a transverse connector increases the allowable length of a pedicle screw and improves pullout strength.[36–38] Also, diverging the screws in the sagittal plane increases axial load-bearing capacity. Furthermore, screws should be aimed toward the stronger subchondral bone near the endplate.[39]

The type of pedicle screw itself can alter fixation. For example, conical screws may be used over conventional cylindrical screws to improve fixation strength.[40,41] However, there is controversy regarding whether backing out the conical screw by 180° or 360° may potentially decrease overall pullout strength.[42,43] Ideally, pedicle screws should be placed at the appropriate depth and should not have to be backed out or reinserted because this decreases insertional torque and pullout strength with any screw.[44] Also, expandable pedicle screws can decrease the risk of screw loosening compared with conventional pedicle screws.[45] Hooks and wires are another fixation option and rely on relatively spared cortical laminar bone and can be used to enhance fixation. One option to use this technique involves using hooks at the cephalad and caudal aspects of the construct.[46]

In the anterior spine, Huang and colleagues[47] analyzed various configurations of double-screw fixation and reported that triangulation of 2 anterior vertebral screws (22° intersection angle) without penetration of the cortex achieved pullout strengths similar to that of 2 parallel double-cortical screws. Although tapping has been shown to improve screw trajectory, undertapping or no tapping with maximization of pedicle screw diameter increases pullout strength and decreases the risk of failure.[48] There was a 47% increase in pullout strength by undertapping by 1 mm compared with undertapping by 0.5 mm.[49] Adding PMMA or calcium phosphate to the screw tract or vertebral body can significantly increase pullout strength.[41,50] The addition of PMMA gives immediate restoration of strength and stiffness and increases pullout strength by 149%.[51] Placement of the pedicle screw while the PMMA is soft increased pullout strength more than placement of the pedicle screw while the PMMA has hardened.[52] Hydroxyapatite-coated pedicle screws also increase fixation and pullout strength.[53] Some surgeons advise vertebroplasty or kyphoplasty at the adjacent levels of a construct to help decrease the risk of fracture. Another technique that can be used is bone marrow aspirate from the vertebral body through the pedicle screw pilot hole to augment the fusion mass; however, bone marrow aspirate used from an osteoporotic spine may not be as beneficial.[54] Meticulous surgical technique involves avoiding in situ correction to seat the rod in the pedicle screw head. This preloading of the screw can weaken the bone-implant interface and cause early fixation failure.

Multiple points of fixation should be used in the osteoporotic spine above and below the apex of any deformity, to achieve a balanced and stable construct.[55] Often, iliac and sacral fixation is recommended to increase fixation strength. In the pelvis, large-diameter screws with bicortical purchase should be used to increase pullout strength.[56] Leong and colleagues[57] showed that divergent S1 screws with use of a Chopin plate (Colorado II sacral plate) increased pullout 20% to 26%. Iliac bar fixation can also be used to augment the distal construct. Fixation techniques simultaneously involving zone 1, 2, and 3 of the sacrum are possible. McCord and colleagues[58] showed an increased maximum stiffness at failure with screw fixation successively from zone 1, 2, and 3. The disadvantage of pelvic fixation is an increased rate of pseudoarthrosis of up to 26% depending on the specific method used.[59]

OSTEOPOROSIS AND SPINAL SURGERY COMPLICATIONS

Multiple complications can occur when operating on patients with poor bone quality. These complications include the risk of neurologic injury, durotomy, infection, wound breakdown, and fixation failure. DeWald and Stanley[60] looked at 47 procedures in 38 patients and found that spinal deformity correction in patients with poor bone quality had an early (<3 months) complication rate of 13%, including epidural hematoma with neurologic injury secondary to pedicle fracture, and adjacent vertebral body compression fracture above and below constructs. They found late complications (>3 months) to include psuedoarthrosis with rod breakage (11%), screw loosening with last instrumented level (7%), acute disc herniation above last instrumented level (4%), pelvic fixation prominence (11%), and progressive junctional kyphosis at the cephalad portion of the construct (26%). However, because of multiple confounders, it is not possible to compare these results of instrumentation-related complications directly with those found in nonosteoporotic patients.

Additional literature suggests delayed union in osteoporotic patients.[61,62] Delayed healing may be due to local osteocytes responding poorly to mechanical stress. In addition, osteoporotic bone has fewer osteoblastic cells present and those osteoblastic cells that are present do not have a normal proliferative response.[63–65] Furthermore, other comorbidities in this patient population places them at increased risk of prolonged intubation and hospitalization.[66,67]

KYPHOPLASTY VERSUS VERTEBROPLASTY

Among the surgical arsenal of compression fracture treatment is kyphoplasty and vertebroplasty. These procedures are generally used for pain relief and to provide structural support for the fractured vertebral body. Vertebroplasty involves the injection of usually PMMA bone cement into the vertebral body through the pedicle to provide structural support. Kyphoplasty involves first using a balloon as a bone tamp to create a void in the vertebral body and restore vertebral height before injection of PMMA to provide structural support.[68] Both kyphoplasty and vertebroplasty result in similar pain relief; however, kyphoplasty allows for a greater increase in vertebral body height and kyphotic angle correction compared with vertebroplasty.[69] One of the most significant complications with these procedures is the leakage of cement and subsequent neurologic injury. The risk of cement leakage depends on many factors, including the specific fracture pattern and cause; however, there is an overall increased rate of cement leakage with vertebroplasty compared with kyphoplasty.[70] There is concern regarding possible compression fracture at the adjacent level of a vertebral body treated with either kyphoplasty or vertebroplasty and long-term studies are needed to better elucidate this potential complication.[71]

SUMMARY

Treating the osteoporotic spine patient involves a multidisciplinary approach with involvement of the primary care physician, endocrinologist, and physical therapist. The spine surgeon should be aware of the unique difficulties encountered while treating this patient population. Preoperative planning is extremely important as the spine surgeon should be aware of potential complications that can occur and various techniques to possibly avoid these complications. Once fusion has occurred, it is important for the patient to continue bone health because adjacent level fractures can occur. With the mentioned concepts in mind, treating the osteoporotic patient can be challenging, but with careful thought and consideration it can be a rewarding endeavor to give patients deformity correction, pain relief, and improved physical function.

REFERENCES

1. Brumback RA. "3.2.1.Impact [factor]: target [academic career] destroyed!": just another statistical casualty. J Child Neurol 2012;27(12):1565–76.

2. Osteoporosis. Available at: http://www.ncbi.nlm.nih.gov/pubmedhealth/PMH0001400/. Accessed July 25, 2012.

3. Prevention and management of osteoporosis. 2003. Available at: http://whqlibdoc.who.int/trs/WHO_TRS_921.pdf. Accessed July 25, 2012.

4. Oleksik A, Lips P, Dawson A, et al. Health-related quality of life in postmenopausal women with low BMD with or without prevalent vertebral fractures. J Bone Miner Res 2000;15(7):1384–92.

5. Silverman SL, Minshall ME, Shen W, et al. The relationship of health-related quality of life to prevalent and incident vertebral fractures in postmenopausal women with osteoporosis: results from the Multiple Outcomes of Raloxifene Evaluation Study. Arthritis Rheum 2001;44(11):2611–9.

6. Silverman SL. Quality-of-life issues in osteoporosis. Curr Rheumatol Rep 2005;7(1):39–45.

7. Kado DM, Browner WS, Palermo L, et al. Vertebral fractures and mortality in older women: a prospective study. Study of Osteoporotic Fractures Research Group. Arch Intern Med 1999;159(11):1215–20.

8. Cranney A, Adachi JD. Corticosteroid-induced osteoporosis: a guide to optimum management. Treat Endocrinol 2002;1(5):271–9.

9. Youness ER, Mohammed NA, Morsy FA. Cadmium impact and osteoporosis: Mechanism of action. Toxicol Mech Methods 2012;18:18.

10. Fini M, Salamanna F, Veronesi F, et al. Role of obesity, alcohol and smoking on bone health. Front Biosci (Elite Ed) 2012;4:2686–706.

11. Zmuda JM, Sheu YT, Moffett SP. Genetic epidemiology of osteoporosis: past, present, and future. Curr Osteoporos Rep 2005;3(3):111–5.

12. Pranic-Kragic A, Radic M, Martinovic-Kaliterna D, et al. Glucocorticoid induced osteoporosis. Acta Clin Croat 2011;50(4):563–6.

13. Tracy JK, Meyer WA, Flores RH, et al. Racial differences in rate of decline in bone mass in older men: the Baltimore men's osteoporosis study. J Bone Miner Res 2005;20(7):1228–34.

14. Cortet B, Houvenagel E, Puisieux F, et al. Spinal curvatures and quality of life in women with vertebral fractures secondary to osteoporosis. Spine (Phila Pa 1976) 1999;24(18):1921–5.

15. Carreon LY, Puno RM, Dimar JR 2nd, et al. Perioperative complications of posterior lumbar decompression and arthrodesis in older adults. J Bone Joint Surg Am 2003;85(11):2089–92.

16. Gennari L, Merlotti D, Nuti R. Selective estrogen receptor modulator (SERM) for the treatment of osteoporosis in postmenopausal women: focus on lasofoxifene. Clin Interv Aging 2010;5:19–29.

17. Lippuner K. Medical treatment of vertebral osteoporosis. Eur Spine J 2003;12(Suppl 2):S132–41.

18. Cheng MH, Chen JF, Fuh JL, et al. Osteoporosis treatment in postmenopausal women with pre-existing fracture. Taiwan J Obstet Gynecol 2012;51(2):153–66.

19. Morris CD, Einhorn TA. Bisphosphonates in orthopaedic surgery. J Bone Joint Surg Am 2005;87(7):1609–18.

20. Huang RC, Khan SN, Sandhu HS, et al. Alendronate inhibits spine fusion in a rat model. Spine (Phila Pa 1976) 2005;30(22):2516–22.

21. Lehman RA Jr, Kuklo TR, Freedman BA, et al. The effect of alendronate sodium on spinal fusion: a rabbit model. Spine J 2004;4(1):36–43.

22. Nagahama K, Kanayama M, Togawa D, et al. Does alendronate disturb the healing process of posterior

lumbar interbody fusion? A prospective randomized trial. J Neurosurg Spine 2011;14(4):500–7.

23. Nakao S, Minamide A, Kawakami M, et al. The influence of alendronate on spine fusion in an osteoporotic animal model. Spine (Phila Pa 1976) 2011;36(18): 1446–52.

24. Lippuner K. The future of osteoporosis treatment - a research update. Swiss Med Wkly 2012;142: w13624.

25. Sinaki M. Critical appraisal of physical rehabilitation measures after osteoporotic vertebral fracture. Osteoporos Int 2003;14(9):773–9.

26. Sinaki M, Wollan PC, Scott RW, et al. Can strong back extensors prevent vertebral fractures in women with osteoporosis? Mayo Clin Proc 1996;71(10):951–6.

27. Wayne PM, Kiel DP, Buring JE, et al. Impact of Tai Chi exercise on multiple fracture-related risk factors in post-menopausal osteopenic women: a pilot pragmatic, randomized trial. BMC Complement Altern Med 2012;12(7):7.

28. Albert TJ, Purtill J, Mesa J, et al. Health outcome assessment before and after adult deformity surgery. A prospective study. Spine (Phila Pa 1976) 1995; 20(18):2002–4 [discussion: p2005].

29. Okuda S, Oda T, Miyauchi A, et al. Surgical outcomes of posterior lumbar interbody fusion in elderly patients. J Bone Joint Surg Am 2006;88(12):2714–20.

30. Glassman SD, Carreon L, Dimar JR. Outcome of lumbar arthrodesis in patients sixty-five years of age or older. Surgical technique. J Bone Joint Surg Am 2010;92(Suppl 1 Pt 1):77–84.

31. Lorenz M, Zindrick M, Schwaegler P, et al. A comparison of single-level fusions with and without hardware. Spine (Phila Pa 1976) 1991;16(Suppl 8): S455–8.

32. Lenke LG, Bridwell KH, Bullis D, et al. Results of in situ fusion for isthmic spondylolisthesis. J Spinal Disord 1992;5(4):433–42.

33. Ryken TC, Clausen JD, Traynelis VC, et al. Biomechanical analysis of bone mineral density, insertion technique, screw torque, and holding strength of anterior cervical plate screws. J Neurosurg 1995; 83(2):325–9.

34. Zdeblick TA, Kunz DN, Cooke ME, et al. Pedicle screw pullout strength. Correlation with insertional torque. Spine (Phila Pa 1976) 1993;18(12):1673–6.

35. Inceoglu S, Ferrara L, McLain RF. Pedicle screw fixation strength: pullout versus insertional torque. Spine J 2004;4(5):513–8.

36. Ruland CM, McAfee PC, Warden KE, et al. Triangulation of pedicular instrumentation. A biomechanical analysis. Spine (Phila Pa 1976) 1991;16(Suppl 6): S270–6.

37. Ono A, Brown MD, Latta LL, et al. Triangulated pedicle screw construct technique and pull-out strength of conical and cylindrical screws. J Spinal Disord 2001;14(4):323–9.

38. Suzuki T, Abe E, Okuyama K, et al. Improving the pullout strength of pedicle screws by screw coupling. J Spinal Disord 2001;14(5):399–403.

39. Horton WC, Blackstock SF, Norman JT, et al. Strength of fixation of anterior vertebral body screws. Spine (Phila Pa 1976) 1996;21(4):439–44.

40. Kwok AW, Finkelstein JA, Woodside T, et al. Insertional torque and pull-out strengths of conical and cylindrical pedicle screws in cadaveric bone. Spine (Phila Pa 1976) 1996;21(21):2429–34.

41. Bai B, Kummer FJ, Spivak J. Augmentation of anterior vertebral body screw fixation by an injectable, biodegradable calcium phosphate bone substitute. Spine (Phila Pa 1976) 2001;26(24):2679–83.

42. Abshire BB, McLain RF, Valdevit A, et al. Characteristics of pullout failure in conical and cylindrical pedicle screws after full insertion and back-out. Spine J 2001;1(6):408–14.

43. Lill CA, Schlegel U, Wahl D, et al. Comparison of the in vitro holding strengths of conical and cylindrical pedicle screws in a fully inserted setting and backed out 180 degrees. J Spinal Disord 2000;13(3):259–66.

44. Defino HL, Rosa RC, Silva P, et al. The effect of repetitive pilot-hole use on the insertion torque and pullout strength of vertebral system screws. Spine (Phila Pa 1976) 2009;34(9):871–6.

45. Wu ZX, Gong FT, Liu L, et al. A comparative study on screw loosening in osteoporotic lumbar spine fusion between expandable and conventional pedicle screws. Arch Orthop Trauma Surg 2012;132(4): 471–6.

46. Hilibrand AS, Moore DC, Graziano GP. The role of pediculolaminar fixation in compromised pedicle bone. Spine (Phila Pa 1976) 1996;21(4):445–51.

47. Huang TJ, Hsu RW, Tai CL, et al. A biomechanical analysis of triangulation of anterior vertebral double-screw fixation. Clin Biomech (Bristol, Avon) 2003; 18(6):S40–5.

48. Erkan S, Hsu B, Wu C, et al. Alignment of pedicle screws with pilot holes: can tapping improve screw trajectory in thoracic spines? Eur Spine J 2010; 19(1):71–7.

49. Kuklo TR, Lehman RA Jr. Effect of various tapping diameters on insertion of thoracic pedicle screws: a biomechanical analysis. Spine (Phila Pa 1976) 2003;28(18):2066–71.

50. Burval DJ, McLain RF, Milks R, et al. Primary pedicle screw augmentation in osteoporotic lumbar vertebrae: biomechanical analysis of pedicle fixation strength. Spine (Phila Pa 1976) 2007;32(10):1077–83.

51. Pfeifer BA, Krag MH, Johnson C. Repair of failed transpedicle screw fixation. A biomechanical study comparing polymethylmethacrylate, milled bone, and matchstick bone reconstruction. Spine (Phila Pa 1976) 1994;19(3):350–3.

52. Linhardt O, Luring C, Matussek J, et al. Stability of pedicle screws after kyphoplasty augmentation: an

experimental study to compare transpedicular screw fixation in soft and cured kyphoplasty cement. J Spinal Disord Tech 2006;19(2):87–91.

53. Sanden B, Olerud C, Larsson S. Hydroxyapatite coating enhances fixation of loaded pedicle screws: a mechanical in vivo study in sheep. Eur Spine J 2001;10(4):334–9.

54. McLain RF, Fleming JE, Boehm CA, et al. Aspiration of osteoprogenitor cells for augmenting spinal fusion: comparison of progenitor cell concentrations from the vertebral body and iliac crest. J Bone Joint Surg Am 2005;87(12):2655–61.

55. Hu SS. Internal fixation in the osteoporotic spine. Spine (Phila Pa 1976) 1997;22(Suppl 24):43S–8S.

56. Ryken TC, Goel VK, Clausen JD, et al. Assessment of unicortical and bicortical fixation in a quasistatic cadaveric model. Role of bone mineral density and screw torque. Spine (Phila Pa 1976) 1995;20(17):1861–7.

57. Leong JC, Lu WW, Zheng Y, et al. Comparison of the strengths of lumbosacral fixation achieved with techniques using one and two triangulated sacral screws. Spine (Phila Pa 1976) 1998;23(21):2289–94.

58. McCord DH, Cunningham BW, Shono Y, et al. Biomechanical analysis of lumbosacral fixation. Spine (Phila Pa 1976) 1992;17(Suppl 8):S235–43.

59. Kostuik JP. Spinopelvic fixation. Neurol India 2005;53(4):483–8.

60. DeWald CJ, Stanley T. Instrumentation-related complications of multilevel fusions for adult spinal deformity patients over age 65: surgical considerations and treatment options in patients with poor bone quality. Spine (Phila Pa 1976) 2006;31(Suppl 19):S144–51.

61. Egermann M, Goldhahn J, Schneider E. Animal models for fracture treatment in osteoporosis. Osteoporos Int 2005;16(Suppl 2):S129–38.

62. Giannoudis PV, Schneider E. Principles of fixation of osteoporotic fractures. J Bone Joint Surg Br 2006;88(10):1272–8.

63. Sterck JG, Klein-Nulend J, Lips P, et al. Response of normal and osteoporotic human bone cells to mechanical stress in vitro. Am J Physiol 1998;274(6 Pt 1):E1113–20.

64. Rodriguez JP, Garat S, Gajardo H, et al. Abnormal osteogenesis in osteoporotic patients is reflected by altered mesenchymal stem cells dynamics. J Cell Biochem 1999;75(3):414–23.

65. Bergman RJ, Gazit D, Kahn AJ, et al. Age-related changes in osteogenic stem cells in mice. J Bone Miner Res 1996;11(5):568–77.

66. Fujita T, Kostuik JP, Huckell CB, et al. Complications of spinal fusion in adult patients more than 60 years of age. Orthop Clin North Am 1998;29(4):669–78.

67. Harris OA, Runnels JB, Matz PG. Clinical factors associated with unexpected critical care management and prolonged hospitalization after elective cervical spine surgery. Crit Care Med 2001;29(10):1898–902.

68. Spivak JM, Johnson MG. Percutaneous treatment of vertebral body pathology. J Am Acad Orthop Surg 2005;13(1):6–17.

69. Liu JT, Liao WJ, Tan WC, et al. Balloon kyphoplasty versus vertebroplasty for treatment of osteoporotic vertebral compression fracture: a prospective, comparative, and randomized clinical study. Osteoporos Int 2010;21(2):359–64.

70. Hadjipavlou AG, Tzermiadianos MN, Katonis PG, et al. Percutaneous vertebroplasty and balloon kyphoplasty for the treatment of osteoporotic vertebral compression fractures and osteolytic tumours. J Bone Joint Surg Br 2005;87(12):1595–604.

71. Boonen S, Wahl DA, Nauroy L, et al. Balloon kyphoplasty and vertebroplasty in the management of vertebral compression fractures. Osteoporos Int 2011;22(12):2915–34.

Managing Atrophic Nonunion in the Geriatric Population
Incidence, Distribution, and Causes

Bryon Hobby, MD[a], Mark A. Lee, MD[b],*

KEYWORDS

- Nonunion • Osteoporosis • Incidence • Etiology

KEY POINTS

- The cause of nonunion in patients with osteoporosis is likely multifactorial, and includes age-related changes in fracture repair as well as challenges in achieving stable internal fixation.
- Age-related changes in signaling and mesenchymal cell function may delay the rate of fracture healing.
- Aged bone cells may have altered responses to the mechanical environment.
- Geriatric patients may use medications that alter fracture repair.
- Locking implants improve fixation in osteoporotic bone and are relevant in nonunion repair in patients with osteoporosis.

Osteoporosis is a systemic disease that affects millions of people worldwide. As life expectancy increases and the population ages, the number of people with osteoporosis is only expected to grow. It is estimated that 50% of women and approximately 20% of men more than 50 years of age will sustain a fragility fracture.[1] As the absolute numbers of fragility fractures increase so too will the absolute numbers of complications including nonunion. Fractures due to osteoporosis often occur in the metaphysis of long bones; common sites include the proximal humerus, distal radius, proximal and distal femur, as well as the spine.[2] The incidence of nonunion in patients with osteoporosis is not well reported in the literature, but failure of fixation for specific fractures is known. Although not all failures in fixation of osteoporotic fractures are due to nonunion, approximate rates can be inferred from these data until studies looking at exact incidences are performed.

Failures of proximal humerus fractures treated with open reduction and internal fixation using a locked implant are reported to be up to 15%. Fixation failure of the distal femur is reported to be 25%.[2] Parker and colleagues[3] showed the incidence of proximal femur nonunion to be 19% in all comers, but the numbers increased as patients increased in age; the rate of nonunion in patients more than 70 years of age was 24.9%. This study did not look specifically at osteoporosis, but those elderly patients are at increased risk for osteopenia or osteoporosis. The same study showed that women are at higher risk of developing nonunion of the femoral neck than men.[3]

The influence that osteoporosis or bone density has on the development of nonunion is debated in the literature. Bonnaire and colleagues[4] recommended consideration of arthroplasty in patients with bone mineral density (BMD) less than 400 mg/cm^3 in displaced femoral neck

a Department of Orthopaedic Surgery, UC Davis, 4860 Y Street, Suite 3800, Sacramento, CA 95817, USA;
b Orthopaedic Trauma Fellowship, Department of Orthopaedic Surgery, UC Davis, 4860 Y Street, Suite 3800, Sacramento, CA 95817, USA
* Corresponding author.
E-mail address: mark.lee@ucdmc.ucdavis.edu

Orthop Clin N Am 44 (2013) 251–256
http://dx.doi.org/10.1016/j.ocl.2013.01.011
0030-5898/13/$ – see front matter © 2013 Elsevier Inc. All rights reserved.

fractures because the decreased BMD would not allow for stable fixation. Hedstrom[5] in a small pilot study showed that those patients with osteoporosis and high levels of bone resorption markers Urinary deoxy-pyridinoline (U-DPD) and serum carboxy-terminaltelopeptide of type I collagen (s-ITCTP) on admission were at increased risk of developing nonunion of the femoral neck. Van Wunni and colleagues[6] showed that BMD had no statistically significant effect on the development of nonunion in patients with fractures who were more than 50 years of age. Heetveld and colleagues[7] found no difference in the rate of revision surgery after internal fixation of the proximal femur between patients with osteoporosis and those without. Animal studies have shown decreased callus formation and decreased bone density in osteoporosis models, but no clear link to nonunion.[8] Age, gender, and accuracy of reduction have been shown to correlate with the risk of nonunion of the proximal femur in several studies.[3,7,9]

Many features of osteoporotic bone lead to increased risk of fracture and make fixation of these fractures difficult. There is an increased cancellous to cortical bone ratio. Cross-linking between trabecular bone is decreased. Cortical bone is more porous and has decreased density, which affects the fixation of implants to the bone. Cellular factors contributing to delayed healing are decreased number of mesenchymal stem cells, decreased number of osteoblasts with increasing age, and impaired response of bone cells in osteoporotic bone cells.[8]

FRACTURE HEALING IN PATIENTS WITH OSTEOPOROSIS

Age-related changes in fracture healing are important considerations in the management of nonunion. Evaluation of the cause of nonunion is uniform across patient populations and includes a thoughtful analysis of the relevant contribution of biomechanical and biological factors. Fracture healing is a complex cascade, which creates significant difficulty in understanding the exact deficiencies or sites of failure in the healing sequence, but stepwise analysis can be helpful in choosing repair techniques.

Changes in Remodeling Potential

In many ways, osteoporosis represents imbalance in bone formation versus bone remodeling. This alteration is potentially problematic for fracture repair as well because efficient fracture healing requires not only new bone formation but also remodeling of callus for appropriate strength. The cell populations involved with remodeling and fracture healing, including osteoblasts and osteoclasts, are subject to cumulative effects of aging that can potentially impair their function. Both glycation and oxidative damage are common in aging tissues[10]; in the setting of cell function, it is likely that these aging processes impair the cell population critical for bone repair.

Local and Systemic Signaling

Age-related changes in the expression of many signaling molecules have been implicated in the process of normal fracture healing, including insulinlike growth factor (IGF) and parathyroid hormone (PTH). Although both IGF and PTH have been demonstrated to increase expression with age, there is no correlation with an improved rate and quality of fracture healing. This finding demonstrates some of the major challenges in understanding the redundant and complicated signaling pathways associated with normal fracture repair.[10,11] Small animal studies show interesting trends. Fractures in old rats are known to heal slowly.[12] In rat defect models, a combination of transforming growth factor β (TGF-β) and IGF-1 together induce healing in critical defect models.[13] Noncritical defect models in aged rats show a similar response to exogenous treatments. Growth hormone applications to healing fractures in old rats can improve bone quality but do not improve the rate of fracture healing to normal levels.[12]

Mesenchymal Stem Cells

Studies on human bone marrow cells indicate that, in a normal host, mesenchymal stem cells can form bone equally well whether from a young or old donor.[14] Clinically, it is observed that bone marrow changes with age and becomes fatty; this evidence is accumulating for several tissues, showing that, with age, marrow stem cells tend to form adipocytes and other cell types. This may become a critical limitation in the application of autologous mesenchymal stem cell harvesting techniques for elderly patients.

Mesenchymal stem cells are rare in adult marrow, and an age-related decrease in numbers has been reported.[15] Although the discreet population of cells that are intricately involved in fracture repair remains elusive, these marrow precursors have been studied extensively in bone models and there is a threshold number of cells required for successful union in both defect and nondefect models (Tseng and Lee, submitted for publication, 2013).

Stem cell senescence related to telomeric shortening has also been studied. Telomerase transfection prolongs the life span of mesenchymal stem cells and enhances osteogenic differentiation and bone formation in mouse models.[16] Age-related senescence of stem cells, which are important for fracture healing, may limit the usefulness of autologous cancellous bone graft harvesting.

Periosteum

Periosteum contains undifferentiated mesenchymal stem cells that possess the potential for chondrogenesis and involvement with the process of normal fracture repair. With aging, the chondrogenic potential of periosteum declines. Periosteum-derived cells from elderly rats respond less well to 1,25-dihydroxyvitamin D_3 (1,25(OH)$_2$D$_3$) and TGF-β than cells from nonelderly donors.[17] Similar findings have been reported in human cells.[18] These studies correlate with the clinical findings of decreased periosteum and periosteal-mediated healing responses in elderly patients.

Mechanobiology

Many of the molecular events in fracture healing are influenced by the mechanical environment, which is sensed by local cells, probably osteoblasts and osteocytes. Bone cells in aged or osteoporotic bone may have altered responsiveness to mechanical stimuli; this has been studied via loading of normal and aged osteoblasts.[19] Differential proliferative potential was seen in osteoblastic cells exposed to cyclic strain from both osteoporotic and normal donors.[20] These findings are a concern because unique fixation algorithms may be required in elderly patients.

Summary

Fracture repair in patients with osteoporosis is likely a unique process. The differences in signaling response, cell populations, and their responsiveness to normal stimuli requires optimization of the biological milieu for successful treatment of nonunion. Approaches used in younger, more optimal hosts may be inadequate in these patients.

PRINCIPLES OF FIXATION IN OSTEOPOROTIC BONE

Surgical treatment of osteoporotic bone depends on many factors including the soft tissues, fracture pattern, and patient factors. The soft tissues in the elderly are often thin and atrophic and certainly at risk for wound complications. Fracture patterns in osteoporotic bone are often comminuted and not inherently stable so this must be considered before surgical intervention. Patient factors such as medical comorbidities and nutritional status must also be considered when planning intervention and to optimize healing. These factors and the principles of fixation must be considered when treating nonunions as well as acute fractures.

Obtaining secure fixation of an implant to osteoporotic bone is often a challenge. With decreased cortical and cancellous BMD, achieving stable fixation in osteoporotic fractures is difficult. The pullout strength of traditional screws is directly related to BMD.[21,22] It is not surprising then that fixation failure in osteoporotic bone is often a result of bone failure rather than implant breakage. Stable fixation in osteoporotic nonunion is made all the more difficult because of the loss of bone stock after hardware removal of the original implant, and the potential increase in bone porosity associated with disuse osteopenia. However, because stable fixation is necessary to achieve a good outcome, much research has gone into implant design and to combat this problem, and this has led to the development of implants such as locked plates and angular, stable, locked, intramedullary nails.

The use of locked plates has improved the treatment of osteoporotic fractures. Locked plates and screws are fixed-angle devices that rely on the interface between the screw head and the plate and function much like an internal fixator. They do not rely on friction between the plate and bone to achieve stability. Individual screw failure is not seen with locked plating, as in conventional plating. Fixed-angle devices resist torsional and angular deformation. Anatomically contoured locked plates also help with reduction and restoring alignment, which leads to more stable fixation. The plate does not have to have intimate contact with the bone, which allows for biologically friendly fixation because the plate can be placed above the periosteum and the blood supply can be preserved.[2,23]

The strategy for surgical fixation should include soft tissue friendly approaches to limit the amount of dissection because the soft tissue envelope can be compromised in elderly patients. Relative stability is recommended whenever possible. The use of a load-sharing device such as an intramedullary nail is less likely to fail than a load-bearing device. In the metaphyseal region, fixation with a buttress plate avoids concentration of forces on a single point and distributes the forces across the plate. Fixed-angle devices are recommended because they resist angular and torsional deforming forces.[1,2,23]

In addition to improved implant design, many investigators have described techniques of augmenting fixation in osteoporotic bone. A commonly described method of augmenting fixation is the use of polymethylmethacrylate (PMMA) around or through screws. This has been shown to increase the pullout strength in many different constructs in osteoporotic bone as well as the spine.[24–28] PMMA has also been used in kyphoplasty for spinal compression fractures.[29,30] One case series of 6 patients reported good results with the use of a PMMA strut in concert with retrograde intramedullary nailing for distal femur nonunions.[31]

Structural bone grafts have also been described in the literature for augmenting fixation in osteoporotic fractures, primarily of proximal humerus fractures. Recently, many articles have reported on results and techniques using an endosteal fibular strut allograft to supplement locking plate fixation with good results in achieving union and decreasing complications.[32–35] Vidyadhara and colleagues[36] reported a series of humeral nonunions treated with an intramedullary fibular autograft and fixation with a dynamic compression plate, achieving union in all 6 patients by 3 months.

The use of bone graft substitutes such as calcium phosphate has also been described to augment fixation in osteoporotic bone. Calcium phosphate has been studied and shown to increase pedicle screw pullout strength in the spine.[37,38] Panchbhavi and colleagues[39] used calcium phosphate to increase screw purchase in an osteoporotic distal fibula fracture model. Gradl and colleagues[40] reported decreased screw cut out and increased axial stiffness in a biomechanical cadaveric model. Calcium phosphate seems to be advantageous in supplementing fixation and has added benefit of eventually being replaced by bone.

PHARMACOTHERAPY

The use of medications in the treatment of fracture nonunion in patients with osteoporosis is poorly studied. The decision to treat patients with nonunions surgically or solely with pharmacotherapy is similar to the treatment algorithms used in patients without osteoporosis. In patients with loss of stable fixation and any resultant or persistent deformity, surgical treatment with deformity correction is indicated. With stable fixation and no significant deformity, symptomatic nonunions may be treated with nonsurgical interventions, including pharmacologic approaches.

Antiosteoporosis Medications

The oldest and probably most common medications are the bisphosphonates, which are antiresorptive medications. These medications target osteoclast function by interfering with remodeling and are, at least, theoretically, a concern in the setting of fracture healing. Experimental studies have shown a larger and stronger callus and delayed remodeling without a delay in the rate of healing. Overall, larger calluses and stronger calluses are seen in most animal models.[41] Clinical use of these drugs is, however, problematic; there are new concerns related to long-term use and the potential association with atypical femoral fractures. Because remodeling is a normal part of the fracture repair process, discontinuation of bisphosphonates should be considered during the fracture repair process.

A human monoclonal antibody to receptor activator for nuclear factor κB ligand (RANKL) has emerged as a new treatment of osteoporosis. The function of this therapy should be similar to that of bisphosphonates and animal studies show similar effects in fracture care with increased callus and delayed remodeling.[41] The effects on fracture healing in humans have yet to be determined.

Anabolic therapies for osteoporosis are interesting and promising for treatment of nonunion. PTH has been studied in several models with both normal and impaired fracture healing.[42] In normal bone, larger calluses are formed at an accelerated rate. In a model of age-impaired fracture healing, high-dose PTH increased the mechanical strength of healing fractures in aging rats (27 months old). Callus formation was delayed in the old rats compared with the young controls.[43] These data are exciting and relevant to nonunion treatment because PTH may be an important tool in preventing the delay in fracture healing caused by aging. However, the clinical use of this product is limited by its cost, narrow indications (necessary for insurance coverage) for osteoporosis, failure of first-line therapies, daily subcutaneous dosing, and protracted treatment times (daily treatment through union and potentially beyond that time point).

Bone Morphogenetic Protein

The effects of bone morphogenetic protein (BMP) in animal models are well described. Clinical application of BMP-7 for recalcitrant nonunion and off-label use of BMP-2 in bone grafting composites have demonstrated good performance and effect. BMP-7 can effectively stimulate fracture repair in both young (3 months) and old (18 months) rats,[44] although the effect on the rate of healing was more significant in young rats. These findings indicate that aging can diminish the response to a therapeutic intervention such as recombinant human BMP-7, nevertheless, geriatric rodents retain their potential to respond to the therapy.

Calcium and Vitamin D Supplementation

Vitamin D deficiency has been implicated in nonunions and this specific deficiency is common in elderly patients with osteoporosis. Several animal studies have shown that vitamin D treatment promotes both fracture healing and the mechanical strength of fracture callus. Human studies are limited but suggest that calcium and vitamin D_3 supplementation could enhance callus formation in patients with osteopenia or osteoporosis.[45] In the absence of significant data regarding the morbidity of standard calcium and vitamin D supplementation, routine prescription during nonunion treatment seem warranted.

REFERENCES

1. Cornell CN, Ayalon O. Evidence for success with locking plates for fragility fractures. HSS J 2011;7(2):164–9.
2. Giannoudis PV, Schneider E. Principles of fixation of osteoporotic fractures. J Bone Joint Surg Br 2006;88(10):1272–8.
3. Parker MJ, Raghavan R, Gurusamy K. Incidence of fracture-healing complications after femoral neck fractures. Clin Orthop Relat Res 2007;458:175–9.
4. Bonnaire F, Zenker H, Lill C, et al. Treatment strategies for proximal femur fractures in osteoporotic patients. Osteoporos Int 2005;16(Suppl 2):S93–102.
5. Hedstrom M, Saaf M, Brosjo E, et al. Positive effects of short-term growth hormone treatment on lean body mass and BMC after a hip fracture: a double-blind placebo-controlled pilot study in 20 patients. Acta Orthop Scand 2004;75(4):394–401.
6. van Wunnik BP, Weijers PH, van Helden SH, et al. Osteoporosis is not a risk factor for the development of nonunion: a cohort nested case-control study. Injury 2011;42(12):1491–4.
7. Heetveld MJ, Raaymakers EL, van Eck-Smit BL, et al. Internal fixation for displaced fractures of the femoral neck. Does bone density affect clinical outcome? J Bone Joint Surg Br 2005;87(3):367–73.
8. Giannoudis P, Tzioupis C, Almalki T, et al. Fracture healing in osteoporotic fractures: is it really different? A basic science perspective. Injury 2007;38(Suppl 1):S90–9.
9. Toh EM, Sahni V, Acharya A, et al. Management of intracapsular femoral neck fractures in the elderly; is it time to rethink our strategy? Injury 2004;35(2):125–9.
10. Carrington JL. Aging bone and cartilage: cross-cutting issues. Biochem Biophys Res Commun 2005;328(3):700–8.
11. Gruber R, Koch H, Doll BA, et al. Fracture healing in the elderly patient. Exp Gerontol 2006;41(11):1080–93.
12. Bak B, Andreassen TT. The effect of growth hormone on fracture healing in old rats. Bone 1991;12(3):151–4.
13. Blumenfeld I, Srouji S, Lanir Y, et al. Enhancement of bone defect healing in old rats by TGF-beta and IGF-1. Exp Gerontol 2002;37(4):553–65.
14. Kirkland JL, Tchkonia T, Pirtskhalava T, et al. Adipogenesis and aging: does aging make fat go MAD? Exp Gerontol 2002;37(6):757–67.
15. Bergman RJ, Gazit D, Kahn AJ, et al. Age-related changes in osteogenic stem cells in mice. J Bone Miner Res 1996;11(5):568–77.
16. Gronthos S, Chen S, Wang CY, et al. Telomerase accelerates osteogenesis of bone marrow stromal stem cells by upregulation of CBFA1, osterix, and osteocalcin. J Bone Miner Res 2003;18(4):716–22.
17. Shiels MJ, Mastro AM, Gay CV. The effect of donor age on the sensitivity of osteoblasts to the proliferative effects of TGF(beta) and 1,25(OH(2)) vitamin D(3). Life Sci 2002;70(25):2967–75.
18. Martinez ME, Medina S, Sanchez M, et al. Influence of skeletal site of origin and donor age on 1,25(OH)$_2$D$_3$-induced response of various osteoblastic markers in human osteoblastic cells. Bone 1999;24(3):203–9.
19. Augat P, Simon U, Liedert A, et al. Mechanics and mechano-biology of fracture healing in normal and osteoporotic bone. Osteoporos Int 2005;16(Suppl 2):S36–43.
20. Neidlinger-Wilke C, Stalla I, Claes L, et al. Human osteoblasts from younger normal and osteoporotic donors show differences in proliferation and TGF beta-release in response to cyclic strain. J Biomech 1995;28(12):1411–8.
21. Chapman JR, Harrington RM, Lee KM, et al. Factors affecting the pullout strength of cancellous bone screws. J Biomech Eng 1996;118(3):391–8.
22. Perren SM. Backgrounds of the technology of internal fixators. Injury 2003;34(Suppl 2):B1–3.
23. Curtis R, Goldhahn J, Schwyn R, et al. Fixation principles in metaphyseal bone–a patent based review. Osteoporos Int 2005;16(Suppl 2):S54–64.
24. Pinera AR, Duran C, Lopez B, et al. Instrumented lumbar arthrodesis in elderly patients: prospective study using cannulated cemented pedicle screw instrumentation. Eur Spine J 2011;20(Suppl 3):408–14.
25. Sawakami K, Yamazaki A, Ishikawa S, et al. Polymethylmethacrylate augmentation of pedicle screws increases the initial fixation in osteoporotic spine patients. J Spinal Disord Tech 2012;25(2):E28–35.
26. Sermon A, Boner V, Boger A, et al. Potential of polymethylmethacrylate cement-augmented helical proximal femoral nail antirotation blades to improve implant stability–a biomechanical investigation in

human cadaveric femoral heads. J Trauma Acute Care Surg 2012;72(2):E54–9.

27. Chen LH, Tai CL, Lee DM, et al. Pullout strength of pedicle screws with cement augmentation in severe osteoporosis: a comparative study between cannulated screws with cement injection and solid screws with cement pre-filling. BMC Musculoskelet Disord 2011 1;12:33. http://dx.doi.org/10.1186/1471-2474-12-33.

28. Unger S, Erhart S, Kralinger F, et al. The effect of in situ augmentation on implant anchorage in proximal humeral head fractures. Injury 2012;43(10):1759–63.

29. Ondul S, Durmus M. Minimally invasive stabilization of vertebralcompression fractures using balloon kyphoplasty. J Neurosurg Sci 2012;56(4):357–61.

30. Phillips FM, Ho E, Campbell-Hupp M, et al. Early radiographic andclinical results of balloon kyphoplasty for the treatment of osteoporoticvertebral compression fractures. Spine 2003;28(19):2260–5.

31. Wu CC. Modified retrograde-locked nailing for aseptic femoral supracondylar nonunion with severe osteoporosis in elderly patients. J Trauma 2011;71(2):E26–30.

32. Bae JH, Oh JK, Chon CS, et al. The biomechanical performance of locking plate fixation with intramedullary fibular strut graft augmentation in the treatment of unstable fractures of the proximal humerus. J Bone Joint Surg Br 2011;93(7):937–41.

33. Gardner MJ, Boraiah S, Helfet DL, et al. Indirect medial reduction and strut support of proximal humerus fractures using an endosteal implant. J Orthop Trauma 2008;22(3):195–200.

34. Matassi F, Angeloni R, Carulli C, et al. Locking plate and fibular allograft augmentation in unstable fractures of proximal humerus. Injury 2012;43(11):1939–42.

35. Neviaser AS, Hettrich CM, Beamer BS, et al. Endosteal strut augment reduces complications associated with proximal humeral locking plates. Clin Orthop Relat Res 2011;469(12):3300–6.

36. Vidyadhara S, Vamsi K, Rao SK, et al. Use of intramedullary fibular strut graft: a novel adjunct to plating in the treatment of osteoporotic humeral shaft nonunion. Int Orthop 2009;33(4):1009–14.

37. Moore DC, Maitra RS, Farjo LA, et al. Restoration of pedicle screw fixation with an in situ setting calcium phosphate cement. Spine (Phila Pa 1976) 1997;22(15):1696–705.

38. Rohmiller MT, Schwalm D, Glattes RC, et al. Evaluation of calcium sulfate paste for augmentation of lumbar pedicle screw pullout strength. Spine J 2002;2(4):255–60.

39. Panchbhavi VK, Vallurupalli S, Morris R, et al. The use of calcium sulfate and calcium phosphate composite graft to augment screw purchase in osteoporotic ankles. Foot Ankle Int 2008;29(6):593–600.

40. Gradl G, Knobe M, Stoffel M, et al. Biomechanical evaluation of locking plate fixation of proximal humeral fractures augmented with calcium phosphate cement. J Orthop Trauma 2012. [Epub ahead of print].

41. Larsson S, Fazzalari NL. Anti-osteoporosis therapy and fracture healing. Arch Orthop Trauma Surg 2012. [Epub ahead of print].

42. Jorgensen NR, Schwarz P. Effects of anti-osteoporosis medications on fracture healing. Curr Osteoporos Rep 2011;9(3):149–55.

43. Andreassen TT, Fledelius C, Ejersted C, et al. Increases in callus formation and mechanical strength of healing fractures in old rats treated with parathyroid hormone. Acta Orthop Scand 2001;72(3):304–7.

44. Hak DJ, Makino T, Niikura T, et al. Recombinant human BMP-7 effectively prevents non-union in both young and old rats. J Orthop Res 2006;24(1):11–20.

45. Doetsch AM, Faber J, Lynnerup N, et al. The effect of calcium and vitamin D supplementation on the healing of the proximal humerus fracture: a randomized placebo-controlled study. Calcif Tissue Int 2004;75(3):183–8.

Index

Note: Page numbers of article titles are in **boldface** type.

Orthop Clin N Am 44 (2013) 257–260
http://dx.doi.org/10.1016/S0030-5898(13)00020-5
0030-5898/13/$ – see front matter © 2013 Elsevier Inc. All rights reserved.

orthopedic.theclinics.com

Moving?

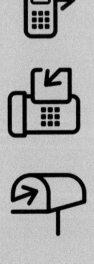

Make sure your subscription moves with you!

To notify us of your new address, find your **Clinics Account Number** (located on your mailing label above your name), and contact customer service at:

Email: journalscustomerservice-usa@elsevier.com

800-654-2452 (subscribers in the U.S. & Canada)
314-447-8871 (subscribers outside of the U.S. & Canada)

Fax number: 314-447-8029

Elsevier Health Sciences Division
Subscription Customer Service
3251 Riverport Lane
Maryland Heights, MO 63043

*To ensure uninterrupted delivery of your subscription, please notify us at least 4 weeks in advance of move.

Printed and bound by CPI Group (UK) Ltd, Croydon, CR0 4YY

03/10/2024

01040344-0009